INTRODUCTION TO
THE NEUROLOGIC
EXAMINATION

INTRODUCTION TO THE NEUROLOGIC EXAMINATION

Michael F. Nolan, PhD, PT

Associate Professor (Anatomy)

Associate Professor (Neurology)

University of South Florida

College of Medicine

Tampa, Florida

F. A. DAVIS COMPANY

Philadelphia

F. A. Davis Company
1915 Arch Street
Philadelphia, PA 19103

Printed in the United States of America

Last digit indicates print number: 10 9 8 7 6 5 4

Medical Editor: Robert W. Reinhardt
Medical Developmental Editor: Bernice M. Wissler
Medical Production Editor: Jessica Howie Martin
Cover Designer: Steven R. Morrone

As new scientific information becomes available through basic and clinical research, recommended treatments and drug therapies undergo changes. The author(s) and publisher have done everything possible to make this book accurate, up to date, and in accord with accepted standards at the time of publication. The authors, editors, and publisher are not responsible for errors or omissions or for consequences from application of the book, and make no warranty, expressed or implied, in regard to the contents of the book. Any practice described in this book should be applied by the reader in accordance with professional standards of care used in regard to the unique circumstances that may apply in each situation. The reader is advised always to check product information (package inserts) for changes and new information regarding dose and contraindications before administering any drug. Caution is especially urged when using new or infrequently ordered drugs.

Library of Congress Cataloging-in-Publication Data

Nolan, Michael, F., 1947–
    Introduction to the neurologic examination / Michael F. Nolan.
        p.   cm.
    ISBN 0-8036-0017-8 (pbk. : alk. paper)
    1. Neurologic examination   I. Title.
    [DNLM: 1. Neurologic Examination—methods.   2. Nervous System—anatomy & histology.   3. Nervous System—physiology.   WL 141 N787i
    1996]
RC348.N65   1996
616.8′0475—dc20
DNLM/DLC
for Library of Congress   95–21837
                                                                              CIP

PREFACE

The human nervous system is an evolutionary product of exceptional beauty and complexity. Its relative importance among the organ systems of the body is suggested by the bony structures in which it is encased and the carefully regulated fluid environment in which it is immersed. These protective measures cannot be viewed as too extravagant if we consider the major functions of the nervous system, which are to regulate and control essential functions and behaviors that are necessary for survival and to provide us with a precise awareness and experience of the constantly changing environment in which we live. Therefore, when disease or injury alters the integrity of the nervous system, normal experience and behavior will certainly be affected, sometimes profoundly. The truth of this statement is not subject to serious debate.

It is generally acknowledged that the first and perhaps the most important task of the clinician is thorough evaluation of patients with complaints of discomfort or disability. The clinician must always recognize and interpret the signs and symptoms of neurologic disease before efforts at therapeutic intervention can begin. In fact, the likelihood of success in treating patients with neurologic disease is directly related to the accuracy and precision of the diagnostic formulation, which in turn is based largely on the results and interpretation of the neurologic evaluation.

The purpose of this book is to provide the reader with an organized and reasoned approach to the conduct and interpretation of the neurologic evaluation. Essential components of the neurologic history and examination are identified and a plan for conducting the evaluation is suggested. Tests and procedures are described, together with appropriate methods for documenting results or observations. Pertinent neuroanatomic and neurophysiologic concepts that form the basis for particular test procedures are also presented, with a brief explanation of how structures and processes govern normal neurologic function. The value of this approach to the neurologic examination is seen in the fact that, if the clinician understands the anatomic and physiologic requirements for normal neurologic function, he or she can more easily and confidently recognize abnormal function.

It is not sufficient, however, to grasp only the neuroanatomic and physiologic bases of individual tests of neurologic function. Nor is it sufficient to acquire proficiency in the techniques of neurologic testing; anyone can be taught to wield a percussion hammer, use a tuning fork, or look into someone's eye with an ophthalmoscope. The clinician must also acquire skill in interpreting test findings. The ability to perform the neurologic examination, even with great skill, is of little value if the clinician cannot interpret the findings and draw reasonable and appropriate inferences. Similar reasoning can be applied to the neurologic history. Most clinicians have little difficulty in asking questions, but skill, sensitivity, and insight are needed to ask the correct ones—questions that will provide useful and important information regarding the nature of the neurologic disorder and the effect it may be having on the patient and his or her family and friends.

It is not the intent of this book to consider the major diseases or causes of disease that produce neurologic dysfunction. These subjects are well covered in standard textbooks on neurology and neuropathology, and the reader is encouraged to consult these books as often as necessary to join the ranks of the learned.

The first part of this book sets forth the goals and objectives of the neurologic evaluation and considers three fundamental questions that reflect the focused purposes of the neurologic evaluation and suggest its overall organization. These questions must be answered for each patient through a correct interpretation of the results of the neurologic history and examination.

The second and third parts of the book, the largest section, deal with these two specific components of the neurologic evaluation, the neurologic history and the neurologic examination. Individual parts of each are identified and described in sufficient detail to enable the reader, who may be studying these topics for the first time, to perform a complete and thorough neurologic evaluation and draw reasoned conclusions from the results. A sequence of activities is suggested as an aid in remembering the various essential components of the evaluation.

Part II identifies specific elements of the neurologic history and suggests their contribution to the development of an accurate impression of the neurologic status of the patient.

Part III details individual components of the neurologic examination.

The proper technique for performing particular tests and maneuvers is presented, and normal and commonly encountered abnormal findings are described. Advice on documenting observations and impressions is included. Some test maneuvers must be performed with special care to ensure the reliability of the observations. The rationale behind these technical and procedural requirements is explored, together with a description of easily made mistakes and common problems in interpretation that may occur if the tests are performed incorrectly.

The Appendices include a form that can be used for making notes while performing the neurologic history and examination and an outline for preparing written or oral presentations of findings. The form suggests an organizational structure for the history and examination that is fairly standard and commonly used in clinical practice. Its use is strongly recommended for the novice clinician to help ensure that the evaluation is complete and that important aspects are not overlooked. The form is comprehensive in scope, emphasizing my belief that students must learn the complete neurologic examination and master its individual components before they can perform and correctly interpret the results of a less comprehensive evaluation.

I hope that the interested clinician, having read this book, will be able to obtain a meaningful history, perform a competent neurologic examination, and correctly interpret and document the obtained findings. It is my further hope that the neurologic evaluation will not be viewed as a mere robotic exercise to be performed by rote, requiring little more than time, a few tools, and a prodigious memory. Rather, this book is intended to make the neurologic evaluation a reasoned, purposeful, and dynamic series of interactions between clinicians and patients, interactions that are wisely chosen and skillfully performed to provide examiners with necessary and meaningful information and patients with comfort and confidence in the health care provider in whom they have placed their trust.

MICHAEL F. NOLAN

ACKNOWLEDGMENTS

This is not the first book to be written on the neurologic examination, nor is it likely to be the last. I hope that my contribution will be seen as an improvement on what has been done before and will serve as part of the foundation for what will be written in the future. If I have been successful in my efforts, it will be because I have learned from those who preceded and taught me. In this regard, I must acknowledge the patient and dedicated efforts of Drs. Robin L. Curtis and F. David Anderson, who guided my early learning in neuroanatomy and made clear to me its central place in clinical neurology. Dr. Leon D. Prockop, Professor and Chairman of Neurology at the University of South Florida, an extraordinary teacher and compassionate physician, mentored and supported me in innumerable ways as I prepared to write and actually wrote this book. His clinical approach and experience as well as his deep insight and concern for patients and the human condition, freely shared, helped me focus and direct my efforts in meaningful and clinically relevant directions. Dr. Peter B. Dunne, a colleague and clinician of remarkable wisdom and wit, made certain that I never lost sight of the joy that comes with helping students learn. Finally, I must acknowledge the day-to-day input I received from the Neurology residents at the University of South Florida. These fine young people helped me over many years to distinguish information that might be considered useful and practical from that which is more likely to be unnecessary and of little value. I am deeply indebted to all of these individuals.

CONTENTS

INTRODUCTION

OBJECTIVES OF THE NEUROLOGIC EVALUATION

Inexperienced clinicians often view the neurologic examination as a complicated series of questions and tests that are difficult to master completely. On coming to the end of the series, these examiners feel no better informed about the patient's condition than before they started; they simply wonder why the patient was not referred to a competent neurologist in the first place. This perception and its attendant frustration may result partly from the teaching of the basic neurosciences as largely divorced from any meaningful consideration of their relationship to the neurologic examination. An appreciation of the details of the structure and function of the nervous system should lead quite logically to an appreciation of the questions and procedures that constitute the neurologic history and examination. It is not unreasonable, and in fact may be desirable, to fashion course work in the clinical neurosciences around the neurologic examination. The utility of such an approach for students in the health sciences is readily apparent from the foregoing discussion.

The neurologic examination is a powerful diagnostic tool. It can be argued without exaggeration or boast that a correct diagnosis can be made in 85 to 90 percent of cases based solely on the information gained from a complete, thorough, and competently performed neurologic history and examination. This is not an unreasonable expectation because the clinician who has an appreciation of the normal structure and function of the nervous system can easily detect any abnormalities. Diseases affecting neurons or their processes in a particular region or regions of the nervous system are characterized by predictable and understandable changes in function. The neurologic examination is the singularly most effective method for accurately determining the location, nature, and extent of neurologic dysfunction in a particular patient.

When confronted with a patient with suspected disease involving the nervous system, the clinician is initially interested in answering three essential questions. The first question is:

1. Is there disease involving the nervous system?

If the answer to this question is yes, the clinician must then seek answers to two more questions:

2. Where is the disease?
3. What is the nature of the disease process?

The neurologic history and examination are designed to provide the answers to these questions.

QUESTION 1: IS THERE DISEASE INVOLVING THE NERVOUS SYSTEM?

Although this may seem like an overly simple question, remember that before any kind of treatment can begin, it is necessary to determine whether disease that requires treatment is present. The clinician must determine whether the patient's complaint is consistent with the information obtained from the neurologic history and examination and whether these findings together suggest structural (organic) or functional (nonorganic) disease of the nervous system. Evidence indicating organic dysfunction will prompt the clinician to characterize the disease further, develop a working differential diagnosis, and implement an appropriate plan of action. If the evidence is inconsistent with the presence of organic disease, the clinician may reassure the patient that nothing is wrong or refer the patient to a psychiatric colleague.

To state the question in a slightly different and more complete way, the clinician is interested in knowing whether the chief complaint and any presenting signs and symptoms point to:

- Injury or disease involving the nervous system directly
- Injury or disease involving non-neural structures or other bodily systems that may in turn be affecting nervous system structure or function
- Neither of the above, but rather complaints and findings fabricated or invented by the patient to achieve some ulterior end or to obtain some benefit

To answer this question, the clinician must have an a priori understanding of what constitutes normal structure and function of the nervous system, an understanding of the normal function of other bodily systems, and most important, an understanding of the variations of normality that characterize human experience and behavior throughout life. Without this knowledge, the clinician will be hard pressed to recognize abnormality in a particular patient.

In neurology, as in other areas of medicine, normality is defined and characterized by a range of behaviors and experiences. A limited understanding of the range of normality can be learned by reading, but a full and adequate understanding can be obtained only from the careful observation of many individuals who are free of neurologic disease. One characteristic that distinguishes truly skilled clinicians from those less experienced is the ability to appreciate the variations of normality in the human population. In other words, an essential requirement for answering the question, "Is there disease involving the nervous system?" is a thorough understanding of the experiences and behaviors that characterize individuals known to be free of neurologic disease.

The answer to this first question usually emerges early in the evaluation process and determines the nature and extent of subsequent interactions with the patient. A lack of evidence of neurologic disease will preclude the need to consider certain therapeutic alternatives. An affirmative answer to this question will lead the clinician to investigate the patient's complaint further and will prompt specific efforts designed to answer the second question.

QUESTION 2: WHERE IS THE DISEASE?

Answering this question is a major objective of the neurologic history and examination. The question is actually composed of several interrelated questions, each of which the clinician must resolve in the process of interviewing and examining the patient.

When information acquired from the neurologic history and examination points to the existence of organic disease, the clinician must determine whether the clinical findings are likely due to disease or injury of nervous tissue directly and only, or are the result of disease processes involving other organ systems, which may secondarily produce neurologic dysfunction. The answer to this question has important therapeutic implications because all body systems are interdependent to some extent.

The clinician must also determine whether the signs and symptoms suggest the presence of widespread disease involving neural tissue or point to a localized site of disease or injury. Put another way, the physician must determine if the clinical findings suggest diffuse neurologic disease, a single anatomic focus of disease, or disease resulting from multiple, reasonably discrete lesions. This question cannot be answered without a thorough understanding of neuroanatomy, neurophysiology, and neuropathology.

If widespread disease of the nervous system is suspected, the clinician must determine exactly where the disease-producing lesions are and what components of the nerve cell or what aspects of its function are affected. For example, the clinician will need to determine whether the disease process involves the axon of a nerve cell or its myelin sheath, or perhaps the metabolic machinery of the cell, which is responsible for the manufacture and maintenance of intracellular organelles as well as for the synthesis of neurotransmitter and receptor proteins.

If localized or focal disease of the nervous system is suspected, the clinician must identify the site of the lesion or disease. In doing so, it is convenient to categorize neurologic disease as being localized to one of several mutually exclusive sites. These sites are listed in Table 1, together with terms commonly used to describe disease processes involving these areas.

If suspected lesions or diseases involve the cerebrum, it is important to determine which hemisphere is involved, which lobe or lobes may be affected by the disease, and whether the lesion is in the cerebral cortex, subcortical white matter, or one or more of the deep nuclear structures.

For suspected lesions or diseases involving the cerebellum, the clinician should determine whether the clinical findings suggest disease involving the cerebellar vermis or the cerebellar hemispheres.

Answers to these questions are essential if the clinician is to arrive at a correct diagnosis. However, one additional question must be answered before it is appropriate to consider treatment strategies.

TABLE 1   *Locations of Neurologic Dysfunction*

Site	Dysfunction
Muscle	Myopathy
Neuromuscular junction	
Peripheral nerve	Neuropathy
Nerve plexus	Plexopathy
Nerve root	Radiculopathy
Spinal cord	Myelopathy
Brainstem	
Cerebellum	
Cerebrum	Encephalopathy

QUESTION 3: WHAT IS THE NATURE OF THE DISEASE PROCESS?

The answer to this question should evolve as information obtained from the neurologic history and examination is organized and weighed in the formulation of the differential diagnosis. An understanding of the etiology of the disease or injury and of its natural course is important in determining a plan of action. Such an understanding is also essential if the clinician hopes to explain the nature of the disease to the patient and his or her family and to provide them with reasonable expectations for the future.

The categories of disease processes that should be considered include:

1. Hereditofamilial
2. Traumatic and post-traumatic
3. Toxic-metabolic
4. Infectious and postinfectious
5. Vascular
6. Degenerative
7. Neoplastic
8. Autoimmune
9. Idiopathic

The neurologic history and examination are the primary and most useful tools available to the clinician for determining the nature of disease processes that alter neural function. Their value in this regard cannot be overemphasized. It is possible, however, that a single definitive answer to this question will not be apparent based on the history and examination and that two or more possible etiologies may seem plausible. Only after the information from the history and neurologic examination have been reviewed will it be appropriate to consider other ancillary tests to aid in formulating the diagnosis.

In summary, in dealing with patients with suspected neurologic disease, the purpose of the neurologic evaluation is to obtain accurate and reliable answers to these questions. The answers serve as the basis for developing an effective treatment plan.

THE NEUROLOGIC HISTORY

In the previous chapter, we identified the purposes of the neurologic evaluation and considered specific questions the clinician needs to answer in order to arrive at an accurate diagnosis. We now consider the process and procedures used to obtain answers to those questions.

The single most important and informative part of the neurologic evaluation is the neurologic history. It is impossible to overemphasize its value. A complete and accurate neurologic history alone will usually provide the knowledgeable clinician with sufficient information to make an accurate diagnosis.

2

TAKING A NEUROLOGIC HISTORY

The neurologic history is essentially a conversation between the clinician and the patient in which the patient provides information about the presenting problems. The role of the clinician is to facilitate the conversation so that the patient can give a complete and accurate account of the problem. The clinician must listen carefully and patiently, continually striving to forge a relationship of trust and confidence.

The neurologic history should be the patient's story, and the information obtained should reflect the experience of disease or dysfunction from the patient's point of view. Patients differ in their ability to relate the details of their problem. Some may be unaware of certain features of their disease or condition or may fail to mention particular problems, believing that they are unrelated to their major complaint. Some may withhold information out of fear of what it might mean or what the clinician might think about them or be compelled to do. Others go on endlessly in their description, highlighting every detail while sometimes obscuring one or more of the important features. Considerable skill and experience are required to lead the conversation without manipulating it or intruding into it unnecessarily. Care must be taken to guard against putting words in the patient's mouth or unduly influencing or altering the patient's description of the problem. The most important characteristics of an adequate neurologic history are accuracy and completeness. Ensuring accuracy and completeness is the major responsibility of the clinician.

There are no shortcuts in conducting the neurologic history. It takes practice and experience to learn how to obtain complete and accurate information from a patient regarding neurologic problems. Yet, if the clinician has not developed a reasonable idea of the nature and location of the disease process after interviewing the patient, additional tests or procedures are unlikely to prove helpful. The purposes of these other tests and procedures, as will be evident later, are to narrow the differential diagnosis and to confirm the diagnostic impression gained from the neurologic history.

Table 2 lists the components of the neurologic history.

CHIEF COMPLAINT

The chief complaint (CC) is the first bit of information obtained from the patient about the presenting problem. It is a description of what the patient experiences or believes to be wrong. Complaints generally fall into one of two major categories: those characterized chiefly by sensory or cognitive experiences that are believed to be abnormal, unpleasant, or threatening, such as pain or dizziness, and those that are marked by disability resulting from a decrement or loss of function, such as weakness or blindness. Initially patients should be permitted to describe the problem without interruption. They should be allowed to include any information that they feel might be pertinent to their problem. The clinician must not end this part of the interview too quickly because initially patients may be anxious about being interviewed and may need a little time to think about different aspects of their problems and the way in which they influence their lives. Moreover, a patient may have several complaints that initially might seem unrelated but later turn out to be important or contributory in some way.

Some patients have difficulty in describing their problems in a way that they feel is satisfactory. The clinician may be tempted to help the patient articulate the problem, but care must be taken to avoid supplying the patient with words or ideas about the problem that might be incor-

TABLE 2 *Components of the Neurologic History*

Chief complaint	(CC)
History of present illness	(HPI)
Past medical history	(PMH)
Pertinent health information	(PHI)
Family history	(FH)
Social history	(SH)
Occupational history	(OH)
Review of systems	(ROS)

rect or inaccurate or that might somehow misrepresent the actual clinical features. Skill and experience are required to avoid introducing features of a problem that are not really present.

The written description of the CC or CCs needs to be sufficiently descriptive to give a clear picture of the problem or problems, and it should be informative enough to guide the clinician through the remaining parts of the neurologic history and examination. A properly formulated CC should include at least the following elements:

1. Specific details regarding the problem
   a. Location (localized, widespread)
   b. Severity and character
   c. Temporal features (onset, frequency, duration, continuous, intermittent)
2. Nature and extent of the disability or dysfunction
   a. Effects on activities of daily living
3. How the patient feels about the symptoms or disability; what are his or her concerns

The CC should be documented in the patient's own words. Resist the temptation to translate symptoms into proper medical terminology, because particular terms may suggest a specific condition or diagnosis that may be misleading or proved incorrect. Additional information should be obtained and considered before coming to a decision about the cause or nature of the problem.

In the beginning of this section, we said that the CC is the first bit of information obtained from the patient. Not infrequently, however, patients are seen who have been referred by colleagues or other health professionals, or who may be seeking a second or third opinion, or both. In many of these instances, a diagnosis or tentative diagnosis has already been made, and the patient may be quite willing or even eager to bring this to your attention. You will not be handicapped if you ignore this information at this time. In fact, you may be better off because you are not likely to become biased by the presumably learned opinion of someone else. Remember that your opinions and conclusions, including your understanding of the CC, should be based on your own findings. You are not examining these patients just so that you can reiterate or refute what someone else has already said.

HISTORY OF PRESENT ILLNESS

Once the CC has been described and is understood to the satisfaction of both the clinician and the patient, it becomes important to develop a chronologic history of events that may have caused or contributed to the patient's problem. These details should produce a more complete picture of the problem. Not infrequently, new details emerge when the problem is considered from a chronologic or historical point of view. Careful questioning can help the patient to recall events or occurrences that might have been forgotten or can give the patient an opportunity to confirm or deny the existence of particular symptoms. Among the issues that should be considered in constructing the history of present illness (HPI) are the following:

1. Date and manner of onset
2. Whether the problem has remained the same over time or has changed for the better or worse
3. Whether any activities, factors, or circumstances worsen or improve the problem
4. Any associated phenomena that might be related to the CC in some way

In developing the HPI, the patient may use words to describe the problem that are unclear. Words such as "numb," "blurred," "weak," "dizzy," or "spell" can have multiple meanings, and time should be taken while interviewing the patient to make sure that you understand what the patient really is describing.

Other sources of information that can easily become incorporated into the HPI are previous consultations. Patients themselves generally bring this information forward. Such information might include laboratory data, neuroimaging reports, and phone calls or letters from referring health professionals and is usually accompanied by a provisional or tentative diagnosis. Caution is recommended when using this information because there are no assurances that the tests were performed properly or that the interpretations are valid. Moreover, there is no need to consider this information at this point in the patient workup.

PAST MEDICAL HISTORY

Neurologic dysfunction can result from disease or injury involving nerve cells only or from disease involving other bodily systems that secondarily affects neuronal function. It is therefore important to obtain a complete and thorough past medical history (PMH) from the patient, particularly if a reasonably sound understanding of the problem has not emerged from the HPI.

The patient should be questioned about previous medical problems and the treatments that were tried to resolve them. Be cautious about accepting diagnoses suggested by the patient for these problems. Records from other healthcare providers who have evaluated or treated the patient may be helpful in developing the PMH.

The patient should be permitted and encouraged to describe whatever he or she might remember about past medical problems. Typically, the patient has not thought about these problems earlier in the history, when attention was focused on the CC and other information he or she believed relevant to the current problem. Moreover, patients may not recognize the relevance of particular past events or medical conditions to their current neurologic problem.

The extent and depth of the PMH vary from patient to patient, but the following issues should be explored in detail:

- Previous injuries or illnesses
- Previous hospitalizations and surgical procedures
- Transfusions
- Medical consultations for other illnesses
- Birth circumstances and childhood illnesses, when appropriate

Details regarding the PMH should be complete, including dates, interventions (if any), and outcomes. Many times, information obtained in the PMH demonstrates its value later during the neurologic examination or the formulation of the differential diagnosis. For example, liver disease or particular vitamin deficiencies can cause a variety of neurologic difficulties. Certain types of heart disease can give rise to emboli, which can become lodged in cerebral blood vessels. Cancer involving the lung and other organ systems can metastasize to the brain and produce significant neurologic dysfunction. It is very important, therefore, to obtain and record a thorough PMH.

PERTINENT HEALTH INFORMATION

Information about factors that may affect a patient's health and well-being is an essential and important component of the neurologic history. Pertinent health information (PHI) with regard to the following concerns should be obtained for all patients:

- Allergies (drug, environmental, food, other)
- Immunizations
- Habits (tobacco, alcohol, abuse of drugs)
- Medications (name, dose, frequency, date started)
- Screening tests (blood pressure, cholesterol, complete blood count)
- Cancer tests (skin, colon, prostate, breast, Pap smear)
- Sleep patterns
- Appetite, diet, eating habits
- Sexual habits and partners

FAMILY HISTORY

A complete family history (FH) is not necessary in every neurologic workup, but it can be the most important part of the neurologic history when certain disease conditions are suspected. A number of neurologic diseases and other conditions are hereditary and may be passed from parent to child. If hereditary illnesses are suspected or thought to be contributory, it will be necessary to obtain a thorough FH. The clinician who is still developing skills in obtaining the neurologic history may chart out the family history using the appropriate symbols and genetic designations.

Some patients may have living relatives with a neurologic disease or may remember a relative now dead who may have had a neurologic or other disease. It is important to inquire about these relatives and to develop as thorough an understanding of their problems as possible. Although firsthand knowledge provided by the patient generally is more reliable than information obtained from others, sometimes information from family and friends may be necessary. Because patients may not associate the particular behaviors of a relative with a neurologic disease, it is important that the clinician help the patient to recall behaviors that may signify a neurologic abnormality. For instance, it may be helpful to ask whether any relatives ever had "blackouts," "spells," or "shaking spasms." By using words familiar to the patient to describe neurologic abnormalities, the clinician can obtain a more complete picture of the FH.

In developing the FH, it is also important to note the present ages of living relatives and the age at death and cause of death of deceased relatives. Sometimes members of the patient's family can be helpful in obtaining this information as well, and their assistance should be sought when there is a question of familial disease.

Sometimes a picture emerges from the FH that raises delicate personal or familial issues. The possibility of consanguinity should not be overlooked when considering the cause of a suspected autosomal recessive condition. Questions regarding paternity may need to be explored or confirmed if a suspected disease is or is not evidenced in a predicted way.

SOCIAL HISTORY

The social history (SH) can provide valuable insight regarding possible causes or consequences of neurologic disease. An inquiry into a patient's SH may include questions about upbringing and relationships with parents and siblings. Information about marital status, children and grandchildren, and educational achievement might also be obtained. If the patient has spent time in a foreign country, the details and duration of these visits should be noted. Details regarding the SH may not always point to the cause of a neurologic problem or even contribute to the differential diagnosis, but they generally provide useful information about the patient as a person and a functioning member of the family and society. Equally useful is information about the effect of the neurologic disease on the patient's sense of wholeness and well-being, particularly as these feelings are expressed through family and social relationships.

OCCUPATIONAL HISTORY

The clinician should always inquire about a patient's work or occupational history (OH). Information pertaining to military experience should also be sought when appropriate. If the patient is an adolescent, questions about school and extracurricular activities can be asked, as well as questions about summer or part-time employment.

The clinician should ask how long the patient has been engaged in a particular occupation and whether he or she has had the same job for a long time or has held a number of jobs of short duration. Inquiries regarding job satisfaction should also be made. The nature of the work should be explored to identify potential exposure to toxic substances, repetitive activities, or tasks that might be considered physically or mentally stressful. It is always worthwhile to inquire about accidents or injuries on the job or other situations that might have necessitated time away from work or a change in work environment.

In addition to providing information that might help to identify the cause of a neurologic problem, the OH can also provide valuable information regarding the consequences of a problem. Many people identify strongly with their work or occupation, and the inability to perform their life's work can have significant emotional and behavioral effects.

REVIEW OF SYSTEMS

Because neurologic dysfunction may result from disease or injury to other bodily systems, it is appropriate to inquire about these systems, keeping alert for reports of disease processes that may secondarily impair neurologic function or that may have resulted from primary disease involving the nervous system. The review of systems (ROS) for patients with suspected neurologic disease is conducted in the same way as it would be for any other patient. A detailed description of the content and organization of the ROS appears in Appendix 1 (pages 185–191). In summary, the areas to include in the ROS include:

- Skin
- Head, eyes, ears, nose, and throat (HEENT)
- Breasts
- Respiratory
- Cardiac
- Vascular
- Gastrointestinal
- Renal and urinary
- Female and male genitalia
- Musculoskeletal
- Neurologic
- Endocrine
- Hematopoietic

When reviewing the neurologic system, you should question the patient about pain, headache, syncope, memory, cognition, disorientation, dizziness, speech, swallowing, seizures, abnormal movements, weakness, sensory changes, mood changes, visual or hearing changes, disturbances of gait or coordination, peculiar odors, difficulties with reading, writing, or comprehension, and sphincter control.

The ROS may reveal nothing, uncover deficits or problems unrelated to the present illness, or yield findings that might be critical in formulating the diagnosis, even though they may seem insignificant or nonproblematic to the patient.

SUMMARY

The neurologic history is essentially a conversation between the patient and the clinician in which the patient describes the presenting problems. The patient must be made to feel comfortable in describing these important and personal details and needs to feel that the clinician is being thorough and purposeful in the collection of information. The clinician must be sensitive to the concerns and feelings of the patient and try to facilitate an openness that will yield a complete and meaningful neurologic history. The clinician must strive to develop a relationship with the patient that inspires trust, confidence, and cooperation.

The neurologic history should give the clinician a reasonable idea of the nature of the problem and its cause. The beginnings of a differential diagnosis should be clear. Once the neurologic history is complete, the clinician can begin the next phase of the neurologic evaluation—the neurologic examination; in this phase, the problems and symptoms described by the patient are more accurately and precisely characterized and the differential diagnosis is refined. For the experienced clinician, the neurologic history should provide a guide to what is likely to emerge from the neurologic examination. The neurologic examination should essentially confirm what the clinician already suspects as a result of the neurologic history. For the student or the inexperienced clinician, these insights will not be immediately evident; they may emerge only after the information from the neurologic history and examination has been put together and thought about as a whole. With experience and practice, the importance of a thorough and complete neurologic history will become apparent, and its value in the evaluation process will be more fully recognized.

THE NEUROLOGIC EXAMINATION

From the neurologic history, the clinician should be reasonably confident in answering the question of whether the patient has a neurologic disease. The history should also provide insight into its location and probable cause and should permit the beginning formulation of a differential diagnosis.

The differential diagnosis at this point may, however, include a number of conditions that might be eliminated with the benefit of additional information. The purposes of the neurologic examination are to characterize further and define more precisely the neurologic problem and to confirm or rule out the presence of specific anatomic or functional deficits. Put another way, the aims of the neurologic examination are to refine the differential diagnosis and to strengthen the diagnostic formulation, both of which are requisites to the development of an appropriate treatment plan.

The conversation between the patient and the clinician continues during this next phase of the evaluation, but now the clinician takes more of a leadership role. During the neurologic examination, the patient is asked specific questions and told to perform specific tasks or maneuvers, each designed to assess the integrity of particular functional systems. The results of these questions and tests provide a much clearer and more complete picture of the patient's neurologic status.

This part of the neurologic evaluation is composed of several parts, *each designed to assess the function of specific neural systems. Five parts are typically considered:*

- *Mental status*
- *Cranial nerves*
- *Motor function, including coordination*
- *Reflexes*
- *Sensory function*

These five parts are detailed in the next five chapters.

CHAPTER 3

MENTAL STATUS

The evaluation of mental status includes assessments of a variety of complex neurologic functions that do not fall neatly into the category of either a motor behavior or a sensory experience. They may be considered fundamental functions in the sense that, if they are disordered, the individual may be significantly disabled and unable to function normally in daily life.

In most cases, the general mental status of the patient will be fairly evident by the time the history is completed. However, a formal evaluation of some aspects of mental status is generally necessary because certain types of deficits may not be readily apparent during casual conversation. Some types of deficits may go unrecognized by the patient, whereas others may be consciously denied. Family members or friends are frequently the first to notice alterations in mental function. Occasionally, deficits revealed by formal examination may call into question certain features of the neurologic history, particularly in patients who display problems with memory or recall. Difficulties with language may make it hard to respond to questions or to follow simple commands during the examination, and alterations in level of consciousness or deficits of attention may influence the degree to which a patient can cooperate with the clinician. It is therefore important to establish an accurate impression of the mental status of the patient early in the examination.

A variety of functions are considered within the framework of mental status. A complete assessment should include tests for those listed in Table 3.

TABLE 3   *Functions Tested in the Assessment of Mental Status*

> Level of consciousness
> Attention
> Orientation
> Language function
> Learning and memory
> Cortical and cognitive functions
> Mood and affect
> Thought content

LEVEL OF CONSCIOUSNESS

Assessment of the level of consciousness is the necessary first step in evaluating mental status. Patients who are not sufficiently alert will be unable to cooperate to the extent needed to continue the examination. Although specific terms are used to describe different levels of consciousness, the degree of alertness is actually a continuum. Nevertheless, several levels of consciousness are traditionally recognized:

1. *Alert:* patient is awake and attentive to normal levels of stimulation. Interactions with the examiner are normal and appropriate unless the patient suffers from some type of psychiatric disorder.
2. *Lethargic:* patient appears drowsy and may fall asleep if not stimulated in some way. Interactions with the examiner may get sidetracked. Patient may have difficulty in focusing or maintaining attention on a question or task.
3. *Obtunded:* patient is difficult to arouse from a somnolent state and is frequently confused when awake. Repeated stimulation is required to maintain consciousness. Interactions with the examiner are largely nonproductive.
4. *Stupor* (semicoma): patient responds only to strong, generally noxious stimuli and returns to the unconscious state when stimulation is stopped. When aroused, patient is unable to interact with the examiner.
5. *Coma* (deep coma): patient cannot be aroused by any type of stimulation. Reflex motor responses may or may not be seen.

Obviously, other aspects of mental status can be determined reliably only in patients who are alert. The chances of obtaining a complete and reliable assessment of mental status are proportionally reduced in patients who are lethargic, and virtually nonexistent in patients who are obtunded, stuporous, or comatose.

A method commonly used to produce arousal in the stuporous or comatose patient is to apply sharp pressure over a bony prominence, such as the sternum, or over a cutaneous nerve, such as the supraorbital nerve as it emerges over the eyebrow from the supraorbital foramen. The patient's response to the stimulus should be carefully noted.

The reticular activating system (RAS) exerts an excitatory influence on the cerebral cortex to maintain the alert state. Neurons located in the reticular formation of the midbrain and pons play a central role in this process. These medially located neurons receive synaptic input from virtually all afferent systems (tactile, thermal, vestibular, auditory, chemical) regardless of whether they use spinal or cranial nerves. Some synaptic input also originates from more rostral structures, including the hypothalamus. The axons of reticular formation neurons course rostrally to synapse in the medial, intralaminar, and reticular nuclei of the thalamus. Ascending projections from these diencephalic nuclei distribute to widespread areas of the cerebral cortex. The RAS provides a background of neural input to the cerebral cortex, which serves to maintain cortical neurons at a basal level of firing consistent with the conscious, awake state. Damage to this system results in a loss of nonspecific excitatory input to cortical neurons, making them less likely to respond appropriately to information transmitted to the brain by way of the more clearly defined tactile, auditory, gustatory, and vestibular pathways. The clinical picture associated with reduced activity of the RAS is a reduction or loss of consciousness.

ATTENTION

Patients can be conscious but not attentive. *Attention* refers to the ability to focus and maintain one's consciousness on a particular stimulus or task without being distracted by other stimuli. Patients who are inattentive will have difficulty in concentrating on tasks, including some of the more complex activities that are part of the mental status examination. It is therefore necessary to assess attention early in the evaluation process because the reliability of the results of other, more complicated tests of mental function is based partly on the ability of the patient to concentrate on the tasks involved.

Attention can be assessed by asking the patient to repeat short lists of objects or numbers. Begin with short lists consisting of two items, gradually increasing to longer lists. Inability to repeat six or more items correctly indicates a probable attention deficit. Caution must be used in interpreting the results of these types of tests because patients with deficits of learning and memory (to be considered later) may perform poorly on repetition-type tasks.

An alternative and perhaps more reliable test of the ability to concentrate involves asking the patient to signal when a particular stimulus is recognized. For example, the examiner may read a list of individual letters in random order and have the patient respond each time a particular letter is heard. The signal letter should appear no less than 10 times in the entire series, with 50 or more letters included altogether. The pace of the test should be such that the patient has time to respond to each test letter. Errors include failing to recognize when the signal letter is presented, or signaling in response to an inappropriate letter. Any errors in a test of this sort may suggest an attention deficit.

A simple screening test is to ask the patient to spell WORLD backward. Attentive individuals can usually perform this task with little difficulty. Individuals who have a problem with maintaining attention may confuse the order of the letters.

ORIENTATION

Orientation refers to the patient's awareness of self and certain realities and facts of the present. The assessment of orientation is composed of simple questions to which the patient is expected to give simple and direct answers. The questions focus on the patient's understanding of who he or she is, his or her present location, and the present time and time passage. We refer to these matters as orientation to person, place, and time. The following questions can be used to assess orientation:

Person:
    What is your name?
    Do you have a middle name?
    How old are you?
    When were you born?
Place:
    Do you know where we are right now?
    What kind of a place is this?
    Do you know what city and state we are in?
    What city or town do you live in?
    What is your address at home?
Time:
    What is today's date?
    What day of the week is it?
    What time is it?
    Is it morning or afternoon?
    What season is it?
    What year is it?
    How long have you been here?

Individuals who are oriented should be able to answer all these questions correctly. We typically refer to degree of orientation by noting whether the patient is oriented to all three domains or to fewer than three. Patients may be described as being oriented "times 3" ($\times$3), "times 2" ($\times$2), or "times 1" ($\times$1). When patients are not fully oriented ($\times$3), it is important to indicate the domain in which they are disoriented. Disorientation to time usually appears before disorientation to place or person, and disorientation to place is evident before disorientation to person. Disorientation to time or place can be related to impairment of short-term memory, so patients who are disoriented to time or place should be carefully evaluated for memory and recall.

LANGUAGE FUNCTION

Language is a means of communication between individuals that uses symbols to convey meaning. The symbols of a language may be pictorial in nature and serve to represent an object or an idea in its entirety, or they may be sounds (phonemes) or visual images (letters), meaningless in and of themselves, that convey meaning when ordered in a particular way and presented to the ear or eye. The English language is composed of phonemes and letters that can be arranged in a specific sequence to represent an object or an idea. When we say that we have acquired language, we imply that we have learned how to use these phonemes and letters to communicate our thoughts and ideas to others and in turn can understand what others wish to convey to us. A cortical function, language is the main and most sophisticated form of communication used by humans. Language disturbances profoundly affect personal interactions and cause significant functional disability.

Language disturbances, known as *aphasias*, must be distinguished from other problems that affect communication ability. For example, they should not be confused with dysphonias and dysarthrias, which are mechanical disturbances of sound and speech production often associated with cranial nerve lesions. *Dysphonias* usually result from lesions that involve the vagus nerve or vocal cords. Patients with dysphonias may sound hoarse or speak with low volume. *Dysarthrias* typically result from cranial nerve lesions or muscle diseases and present as difficulties with resonation or articulation. Dysarthrias are not associated with lesions involving cortical association neurons.

Language is used in two different ways: to convey information to others and to receive information from others. Most people perform these functions by speech and writing. (Individuals who are blind may use the sense of touch as a means of receiving information.) It is therefore important to test each of these methods of language use. It is preferable to evaluate speech language before considering reading and writing ability.

When evaluating language function, it is important to pay particular attention to several aspects: spontaneous speech, fluency, comprehension, repetition, naming and word finding, and reading and writing.

Spontaneous Speech

Spontaneous speech can easily be evaluated while obtaining the neurologic history. During this time, the patient both formulates and expresses thoughts and responds to a variety of questions. Patients who demonstrate reduced or absent speech may suffer from dysarthria, aphasia, diffuse brain disease, or one of a variety of psychiatric conditions. Disorders of spontaneous speech, characterized by impairment of the rhythm, pace, or inflection of normal speech (*dysprosody*), may be evident during casual conversation.

Fluency

Fluency in speech is characterized by word flow that is free from pauses or breaks. By this point in the neurologic evaluation, the clinician should have a reasonable idea of the fluency of speech, but if some question remains, fluency can easily be tested by asking the patient to say as many words as he or she can within 60 seconds that begin with a particular letter of the alphabet. The clinician should count these words, noting any repeated words or errors. Patients who produce 12 words or less during 60 seconds can be considered dysfluent. Some caution is necessary, however, in interpreting the results of this type of testing in patients who have limited formal education or for whom English is a secondary or newly acquired language.

Lesions involving the left inferior frontal gyrus, or areas 44 and 45 of Brodmann (Fig. 1), frequently result in dysfluency, particularly in right-handed individuals. The speech of such patients is characterized by articulatory struggle and the predominant use of nouns and verbs. Speech lacks the normal complement of prepositions and other grammatically appropriate and useful words that give flow to spoken communication. Terms frequently used to refer to this condition include *expressive aphasia, Broca's aphasia, motor aphasia*, and sometimes *anterior aphasia*.

Two other forms of dysfluency are stuttering and stammering. They are not forms of dysarthria, dysphasia, or verbal apraxia and can be distinguished clinically from these conditions. *Stuttering* is characterized by difficulty in uttering the first phoneme or sound at the beginning of a conversation. The jaw and mouth may move, but no meaningful sound emerges for some period of time, as if the patient is having difficulty in getting air to pass through the glottis. *Stammering* is characterized by the repetition of phonemes at the beginning or during the course of speech

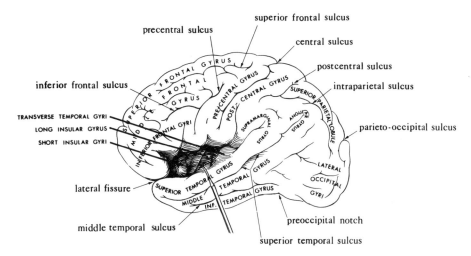

FIGURE 1. Lateral surface of left cerebral hemispheres. (From Dunkerley, GB: *A Basic Atlas of the Human Nervous System.* FA Davis, Philadelphia, 1975, p. 104, with permission.)

that interferes with its normal flow and rhythm. The distinction between these two types of dysfluency may be subtle and of limited clinical value. The cause or causes of stuttering and stammering are not well understood. They may appear spontaneously or after brain injury. When present, they can be detected during casual conversation. In some patients, they can be exacerbated by stress.

Comprehension

Comprehension refers to the ability of the patient to understand or ascribe appropriate and correct meaning to words and sentences. Comprehension can be tested by asking the patient to answer a series of simple yes-or-no questions. At least 8 to 10 questions should be asked, because the chance of guessing correctly is relatively high. Patients with intact comprehension ability should answer all questions correctly. A simple test of comprehension is to ask the patient the following question: "Is my sister's brother a woman or a man?" An alternative test is to ask the patient the following three questions:

"Do you know what a lion is?"
"Do you know what a dog is?"
"If I told you the lion killed the dog, which animal died?"

Patients who have impaired comprehension may demonstrate well-articulated and perfectly fluent speech patterns, but their utterances may be completely out of context or devoid of appropriate content. Comprehension deficits may be seen in patients with lesions involving Wernicke's area in the posterior part of the superior temporal gyrus on the left or the immediately underlying white matter (see Fig. 1). Terms frequently used to describe impairment of language comprehension include *receptive aphasia, Wernicke's aphasia, sensory aphasia,* and sometimes *posterior aphasia.*

Repetition

Repetition is the ability to repeat single words or short lists of words without error. In some patients, the ability to repeat will be impaired even though speech fluency and comprehension are intact. Testing for repetition ability should occur after tests for fluency and comprehension, to ensure that a problem with repetition is not due to impairment of one of these other functions.

Testing should begin with simple monosyllabic words, working to multisyllabic words, then to short series of 2 or 3 words, and ending with longer series of 8 to 10 words. Word deletions, additions, or substitutions indicate difficulty with repetition. For example, an easily administered repetition task would involve asking the patient to repeat each of the following in order (one at a time):

Dog.
Thirteen.
Washington, D.C.
The door is closed.
All the children went to school.
No ifs, ands, or buts.

Although this test is useful in assessing repetition deficits, caution is necessary when interpreting the findings, because patients with attention deficits or disorders of learning and memory may also have difficulty with this task.

Difficulties with repetition result from lesions involving the arcuate fasciculus on the left side. The arcuate fasciculus is a phylogenetically new subcortical association bundle that interconnects Wernicke's area with Broca's area. ~~Brodman's 21 + 22~~

Naming and Word Finding

We learn a language initially by associating auditory symbols (phonemes put together as words) with the objects they are meant to represent. With time, we learn about a great many objects and become able to distinguish between them by the sound of the words used to represent them. The names of most things we learn about are characterized by their unique and distinctive sound. Only much later do we learn how to recognize and distinguish objects and communicate by means of visual symbols (that is, letters).

The ability to name objects is one of the fundamental operations necessary for using language to communicate. Communication between persons would therefore be severely impaired by an inability to name objects or retrieve from memory words that represent objects.

Tests for naming and word-finding ability require patients to supply the names for simple objects they are shown. The patient is instructed to name the object to which the clinician points. Objects used to test naming and word-finding ability should be common everyday objects that virtually any patient would be expected to recognize and with which he or she preferably has some experience. Objects should be of different types and ordered in increasing levels of difficulty. The following categories and objects can be used to test naming and word-finding ability:

Body parts:
  Eye, leg, hand, ear, shoulder, fingernail
Clothing:
  Shirt, shoe, necktie, collar, button
Objects:
  Pen, watch, coin, safety pin
Parts of objects:
  Watch band, belt buckle, watch crystal

Patients with normal naming and word-finding ability should correctly identify all objects presented. Patients who have difficulty may correctly identify body parts or items of clothing but may be unable to name objects or parts of objects. To compensate for their inability to name an object, some patients may launch into a description of the visual characteristics of the object or describe how it is used or what it is used for. Difficulty with naming and word finding is a common finding in patients with aphasia.

Reading and Writing

Reading and writing are means of communication that require language and the ability to use language. The ability to read and write is an acquired skill that is specific to language.

The skill with which a neurologically intact individual is able to read and write is a function of educational experience and practice, so that tests of reading and writing ability are only of value in individuals who have at one time learned these skills.

To test reading ability, the patient should be given a simple text and asked to read aloud. A newspaper or a magazine can be used for this purpose. The clinician should listen to the pace and speed of the reading and note any word omissions, substitutions, or additions. The clinician should also ask the patient simple questions about the text material, to ascertain whether the patient comprehends or understands the meaning of the text. Patients with receptive (Wernicke's) aphasia may have difficulty in reading aloud and with reading comprehension. Patients with expressive (Broca's) aphasia may have difficulty in reading aloud but no problem with comprehension. Patients that have no aphasic problems but are unable to comprehend what they read are referred to as *dyslexic*.

To test writing ability, ask the patient to write or print letters, numbers, words, or sentences in response to your requests. The tasks should be of increasing difficulty and not exceed the level of the patient's previously known or premorbid ability. Word substitutions, additions, or omissions, significant misspellings, or errors in grammatical construction may be evident in the written work. *Agraphia* refers to a disturbance of writing ability in an individual who was previously able to write.

Disturbances of reading and writing are generally associated with lesions involving the cerebral cortex and subcortical white matter of the posterior temporal and anterior occipital lobes of the left hemisphere. Some patients, however, may demonstrate large lesions in neuroimaging studies but display little functional disability on clinical testing.

Because of differences in the extent to which individuals use reading and writing to communicate, disability associated with lesions involving these areas of the brain can vary. For those who depend on reading and writing skills for their livelihood, such a loss can have a profound impact, affecting not only their ability to work but also their sense of wholeness and psychologic well-being.

LEARNING AND MEMORY

Disturbances involving the ability to learn new things for future use and to remember things from the past can have profound effects involving not only the patient but also his or her family, friends, and coworkers. Deficits in learning and memory can be associated with both organic and nonorganic diseases of the brain. The clinical presentation can range from the profound, which is usually obvious to the observer and quite disabling to the patient, to the subtle, which may be evident for only certain types of recall and may not even be recognized or appreciated by the patient.

We will first define some terms and refine our understanding of the processes involved in learning. This brief discussion will serve as a guide to some simple tests that can be used clinically to evaluate these more complex functions.

Learning can be defined as a process that results in a change in behavior as a result of experience. There are recognized molecular and cellular indices of learning as well as behavioral correlates that involve the individual as a whole. In clinical neurology, we are interested mainly in learning at the behavioral level, particularly as it influences the ability of the patient to function effectively in society. Two forms of learning are generally recognized: nonassociative and associative. *Nonassociative learning* involves a change in the intensity or strength of a learned response to an unchanging stimulus. Habituation and sensitization are two types of nonassociative learning. In habituation, there is a decrement in the behavioral response to repeated presentations of the same stimulus. We use the word "extinction" to describe this reduced responsiveness to stimulation. Sensitization is characterized by an enhanced response to repeated presentations of the same stimulus after delivery of a novel or facilitating stimulus. The difference in behavioral response to rubbing the skin before and after sustaining a second-degree burn is an example of sensitization.

Associative learning is characterized by behavior produced by a stimulus or event that did not produce that behavior before learning. Pavlovian conditioning is a classic example of associative learning. Most of the learning that characterizes human behavior is associative learning, and it is this type of learning that we are generally most interested in when we suspect that patients may be suffering from some type of learning disability.

Memory is the ability to recall information or experience from the past. Different types of memory can be distinguished based on the nature of the information stored or the time that has passed between memory acquisition and recall. When considering memory based on the nature of information stored, we can distinguish between declarative and nondeclarative forms of memory. *Declarative memory* is memory for facts and events. It is commonly and easily tested in the clinical setting, as will be discussed below. *Nondeclarative memory* is memory for skills and procedures. It is also easily tested clinically, and indeed may be partially tested when assessing language function.

Short-term memory and long-term memory are distinguished by the length of time that has passed between acquisition and recall. *Short-term memory* is evidenced by the ability to recall information acquired seconds to minutes beforehand. *Long-term* memory refers to the ability to remember and recall information acquired days to months to years earlier. Memory deficits can be specific to either short-term or long-term memory and can be distinguished by clinical examination.

Learning and memory depend on the integrity of the hippocampus and amygdaloid nucleus. Lesions involving these structures or their interconnections with other brain regions can produce very specific deficits in learning and memory. *Amnesias* are memory deficits that are characterized by difficulties in remembering. They can be specific for recently acquired information or for information acquired long ago. Amnesia can be associated with a specific event such as head trauma. Memory deficits associated with head trauma can be specific for experiences occurring subsequent to the injury (anterograde amnesia), preceding the injury (retrograde amnesia), or a combination of both.

Immediate recall, short-term memory, and long-term memory can each be tested in the neurologic examination. However, patients with attention deficits or disorders of language function may be difficult to evaluate. It is therefore wise to delay this testing until the patient's level of attention and language ability have been evaluated.

Immediate recall can be assessed by asking the patient to repeat a short story read by the examiner. Such a story might be as follows:

> After the family packed the car for their vacation, they took their pet dog Midas to their neighbor's house, where he would stay until they returned 2 weeks later. Mrs. Jones drove to the gas station, where they filled up the car with gas and put air in the tires before heading to a ski lodge in the Rocky Mountains.

Patients with normal immediate recall ability should be able to repeat the story, recalling at least half of the details correctly.

A simple test of short-term memory involves presenting the patient with a short list of words and asking him or her to repeat the words a few minutes later. Words representing three unrelated objects should be used. It is necessary to have the patient repeat the words immediately after presentation to ensure that he or she has indeed heard and recognized the words and understood the instructions. Examples of test items are as follows: glove, automobile, orange.

Individuals with no deficit in learning or short-term memory should be able to recall and repeat all three words 5 minutes after presentation and at least two of the words after 30 minutes. Failure in this simple test can be interpreted as indicating a short-term learning deficit.

Visual memory should be tested in any patient with a suspected memory deficit. The test is performed by showing the patient three common, easily recognized objects and asking him or her to remember these items. Keys, coins, pencils, and other common objects are useful for this purpose. After the patient looks at the items for several seconds, the three items are placed in various parts of the room, out of the patient's immediate attention but not hidden. Approximately 5 to 10 minutes later, the patient is asked to retrieve each of the objects and return them to the examiner. Normal individuals should be able to find each of the test objects. Patients who fail to find one or more of the objects should be asked to name each of the items used. Failure to retrieve a test object is usually a result of not remembering what the test item was.

Long-term or remote memory can be tested by asking the patient to recall persons or events from the past. Questions about the patient's own past can be asked, if you can verify the accuracy of the responses given. Specific questions might include:

Where were you born?
What schools did you attend?
In what towns were the schools?
Were you in the military service?
When were you there and what did you do?
Were you or are you now married?
When did you get married?

A better way of assessing long-term memory may be to ask the patient questions of a general-knowledge nature. Specific questions must be appropriate to the patient's intellectual ability, educational accomplishments, and experiential background, however. These questions can be of almost unlimited variety and can be chosen for each particular patient. Questions frequently used for this purpose include:

Can you name any U.S. presidents since you were a young person?
Do you remember which president was shot in 1963?
Can you name any of the wars the United States fought in during your lifetime?

Questions about hobbies or special interests or work-related topics may be asked if it is known that the answers would require information that was acquired a long time ago.

Based on the results of these various tests, the clinician should be able to make a reasonable judgment as to the status of the patient's ability to learn and remember. Pure deficits of learning and memory usually indicate lesions in the temporal lobe specifically involving the hippocampus and nearby amygdaloid nuclear complex. A particular deficit can be generalized or specific with regard to subject matter, transient or permanent in terms of its course, or of gradual or sudden onset, as might be seen following head trauma. From a behavioral and clinical perspective, learning and memory deficits can be relatively mild, producing limited disability, or devastating in their effect, leaving the patient incapable of functioning independently.

CORTICAL AND COGNITIVE FUNCTIONS

Much of what characterizes human behavior and distinguishes one individual from another is a consequence of neuronal activity of the cerebral cortex. Although a variety of behaviors can occur in the absence of a cerebral cortex, most of these are automatic or reflexive in nature and do not reflect the diverse adaptive capabilities of human beings. Damage to the cerebral cortex or the white matter immediately beneath it might therefore be characterized by specific deficits that involve functions and abilities that are uniquely human. We now consider some of these special, cortex-dependent functions and abilities, together with a few simple methods of evaluating them.

Fund of Knowledge

A patient's fund of knowledge is the sum of his or her learning and experiences in life. This knowledge is extraordinarily varied, ranging from knowledge acquired by means of formal training and education to that learned by experience. Everyone's fund of knowledge is different in breadth, depth, and content. When evaluating the fund of knowledge, it is helpful to have an idea of the patient's premorbid knowledge base. Such information greatly facilitates judgments as to whether there has been a decline in mental function from some previous level. Unfortunately, this information is not always readily available. In such instances, an individual's fund of knowledge—at least in some general categories of information—can be reliably determined by careful testing.

Certain conditions must be present or assumed before the fund of knowledge can be reliably determined. It must be established, for example, that the patient is alert, attentive, and not suffering from disturbances of language function or learning and memory. The presence of such problems could hinder an assessment of the fund of knowledge, making the results unreliable. Tests used to evaluate these requisite functions, particularly tests for language function and learning and memory, presuppose some functional level of knowledge. The results of these tests should therefore provide the clinician with at least some idea of a patient's fund of knowledge. Additional testing may be required if a more accurate assessment of this cortical function is necessary. Questions that might be used to evaluate the fund of knowledge include the following:

Who became president of the United States after Kennedy was shot?
Who is the current vice president of the United States?
Which is more—a gallon or a liter?
In what country is the Great Pyramid?
What would you add to your food to make it sweeter?
In what state would you find the city of Chicago?
From where do the space shuttles take off?
What are the elements that make up water or salt?
Can you name a car made by General Motors?
Who is Charles Dickens?

At least 8 to 10 questions of this depth and diversity should be asked. They should not represent areas of knowledge or degrees of difficulty with which the patient is unlikely to be familiar. Nor should they be so simple that they do not give the examiner some indication of the patient's factual fund.

Calculation Ability

The ability to calculate at some level of complexity is acquired by most individuals, even those who are illiterate. The inability to calculate (acalculia) or demonstrable difficulty in performing calculations (dyscalculia) is seen in lesions involving the cerebral cortex, although the localizing value of this finding is not great. Deficits can be identified by means of oral or written testing.

Oral testing involves having the patient perform simple computations involving addition, subtraction, multiplication, and division. The patient should be asked to provide the answers to simple arithmetic questions asked by the examiner. Addition and subtraction are simpler forms of computation than multiplication and division and should therefore be tested first. Calculations involving single digits should be tested before moving to calculations involving multidigit numbers. A commonly used calculation task is "serial 7s," a test in which the patient is asked to subtract 7 from 100, subtract 7 from the remaining number, and so on.* Normal individuals may be slow in performing serial 7s, but they should nonetheless be able to provide the correct responses.

Calculation ability can also be tested in writing. The patient is presented with simple arithmetic problems on paper and is asked to write the answer to the problem below the problem. Again, simple problems should be presented before complex problems. Some examples that might be used in written testing are as follows:

$$
\begin{array}{ccccc}
6 & 11 & 32 & 48 & 27 \\
+4 & +4 & +16 & +26 & +98 \\
\hline
\end{array}
$$

$$
\begin{array}{ccccc}
9 & 16 & 29 & 33 & 91 \\
-3 & -4 & -13 & -17 & -58 \\
\hline
\end{array}
$$

$$
\begin{array}{cccc}
3 & 26 & 30 & 106 \\
\times 2 & \times 5 & \times 12 & \times 48 \\
\hline
\end{array}
$$

The examiner must remember that the ability to calculate is a learned ability and closely related to education level. Interpretation of the results

---

*For examiners like this author, who may themselves have some difficulty with calculations, the correct responses to serial 7s are 93, 86, 79, 72, 65, 58, 51, 44, 37, 30, 23, 16, 9, 2.

of calculation testing must take into account the level of education and premorbid ability of the patient.

Proverb Interpretation

The ability to grasp the meaning of so-called proverbs is a rather sophisticated cortical exercise. It involves not a literal reading and understanding of the words of the proverb, but rather an interpretation of the words, giving rise to a different or new meaning. The ability to interpret proverbs involves learning and memory but requires more than the simple retrieval of past experience. It involves a synthetic process in which new meanings and realizations are derived from previous experience. In testing the ability to interpret proverbs, patients should be asked to explain in their own words the meaning of the proverb. Deficits in the ability to interpret proverbs are associated with cortical disease but have little precise localizing value. Some simple proverbs that can be used to test this ability are:

A stitch in time saves nine.
The early bird catches the worm.
The dog that trots about finds the bone.
A nod is as good as a wink to a blind horse.
The empty wagon makes the most noise.

Gnosia and Agnosia

Gnosia, in general terms, is the ability to recognize stimuli applied to the body. The *agnosias* are acquired conditions characterized by the inability to *recognize* stimuli in the absence of disease involving the anatomic and neural structures involved in transduction, transmission, and perception of those stimuli. (Structures necessary for these processes include sensory receptors of all types, peripheral nerves, peripheral nerve cell bodies, spinal and brainstem neurons involved in the ascending transmission of "sensory" impulses to the thalamus, thalamic neurons that project to the cerebral cortex, and neurons located in the primary sensory areas of the cerebral cortex [i.e., postcentral gyrus, primary visual cortex, primary auditory cortex].) Patients with agnosias have normal ability to perceive a stimulus but lack the ability to recognize the stimulus for what it is. These patients have difficulty in ascribing meaning or significance to particular sensory experiences.

The agnosias can involve any of the five senses. In clinical practice, gnosia testing is usually limited to testing for visual, tactile, auditory, and olfactory recognition, although testing for gustatory recognition is possible.

Testing for visual agnosia is performed by asking patients to identify objects from pictures. The pictures must show objects with which the patient has some familiarity, such as common household objects or items of clothing. Letters, words, and numbers should not be used because they are symbols of language rather than representations of objects themselves. The clinician should keep several small cards with pictures or drawings of these objects available for use in testing for visual agnosias. Deficits of this type may be seen in patients with lesions involving the visual association areas of the occipital lobe (areas 18 and 19).

Auditory gnosia is evaluated by presenting the patient with sounds that might be produced by common objects. For example, the examiner may tap on a drinking glass, close a door, drop a coin on a hard surface, or ring a small bell and ask the patient to identify the sound. The sound must be something the patient has heard before and would be expected to recognize on hearing it again. It may be necessary to present the auditory stimulus several times. Care must be taken to avoid providing the patient with any other sensory cues or information that might provide him or her with the correct answer. Auditory agnosias may be present in patients with lesions involving the auditory association areas of the temporal lobe (areas 42 and 22).

Tactile gnosia is generally tested in two ways. The first testing method involves scribing a number or letter in the palm of the patient's hand (out of sight) and asking the patient to identify the number or letter written (graphesthesia). The second test involves asking the patient to identify a small object, such as a coin, key, or safety pin, placed in his or her hand. Objects should be small enough to be identified with one hand and should not emit any noise or odor that might give a clue as to their identity. The test should be done with each hand separately and should not involve the same object for both hands. Tactile agnosias (astereognosis) may be seen in patients with lesions involving the tactile association areas located in the parietal lobe (areas 5 and 7). Tests for tactile gnosia are usually performed later, during the sensory part of the neurologic examination.

Olfactory gnosia is usually evaluated during testing of the first cranial nerve. A common, non-noxious olfactory stimulus such as coffee or oil of wintergreen or of oranges is presented to each nostril separately. The patient is asked simply to identify the stimulus. The ability to recognize olfactory stimuli is thought to be a function of olfactory association cortices located in the rostral part of the temporal lobe.

Finger agnosia refers to the inability to recognize one's own fingers or those of the examiner. It can be tested using either auditory or tactile stimuli. When auditory stimuli are used, the patient is asked to point to a particular finger on his or her own hand or on the hand of the examiner. When tactile stimuli are used, the patient is asked to close his or her eyes. The examiner then touches a particular finger on the patient's hand, then asks the patient to open his or her eyes and point to or touch the same finger on the examiner's hand. This type of testing can also be used with the toes. Finger agnosia may be seen in lesions involving the parieto-occipital area of the brain.

Praxis and Apraxia

Praxis refers to the carrying out of an action. *Apraxias*, therefore, are characterized by an inability to perform motor behaviors. Specifically, the apraxias are acquired disorders of learned movements that are present in the absence of disease involving the "motor systems" or skeletal muscle. The term *motor systems* in this definition refers to cortical and brainstem upper motor neurons and their axons, neurons of the basal ganglia, cerebellum and brainstem, lower motor neurons and their axons, and skeletal muscles including the neuromuscular junction. Also intact are afferent and ascending systems that convey sensory stimuli to the brain. Thus, apraxias are a type of movement disorder seen in patients who are alert, attentive, and cooperative and have no evidence of disordered strength, coordination, or comprehension.

When testing a patient for a suspected apraxia, first establish, at least in a preliminary way, that the motor and sensory systems are intact. It is also essential to establish that the patient has normal language function and comprehension ability because movement deficits and disabilities that may be seen in patients with communication disorders are different and distinct from those recognized as the apraxias. Patients with apraxic disorders can be viewed as having difficulty with motor planning rather than with motor execution.

Apraxias are sometimes distinguished on the basis of the complexity of the movement or behavior that is disordered. The inability to perform simple one- or two-step motor behaviors is sometimes referred to as an *ideomotor apraxia*, whereas difficulty with the performance of multistep behaviors requiring that movements be performed in a particular sequence is frequently referred to as *ideational apraxia*. Apraxias can also be regional, depending on the part or parts of the body involved. The terms *buccofacial*, *limb*, and *truncal* are commonly used to describe various types of apraxias.

Clinical testing should begin with simple movements and progress to the more complex. Buccofacial, limb, and truncal movements should each be tested separately. The examiner should ask the patient to perform a particular movement or carry out a simple movement task. The following simple motor requests can be used to assess buccofacial, limb, and trunk movements:

Buccofacial:
　Can you whistle a little tune?
　Can you touch your tongue to your upper and lower lips?
Limb:
　Can you show me how you shake hands?
　Can you show me how to use a toothbrush?
　Can you show me how to clap your hands?
　Can you show me how to kick a ball?
Trunk:
　Can you show me how to take a bow?
　Can you show me how to swing a baseball bat?

Some patients may fail in these simple tasks. The clinician may then perform the task, asking the patient to imitate it. Performance may improve in some patients, but the ability to initiate movements does not rule out the existence of an apraxia.

Multistep tasks should be explained slowly and clearly so that the patient fully understands all of the commands. The clinician may even ask the patient to repeat the request to be certain the patient has heard it and comprehends it. One example of a multistep task requires the use of three small bottles with screw tops, one of which contains four white marbles and four black marbles. The patient is instructed: "Take the marbles out of the bottle and place the black marbles in one bottle, the white marbles in the other, and then put the tops back on all the bottles."

Apraxias are most frequently seen in patients with lesions involving the parietal lobe on the dominant side, although lesions in other locations, particularly the left frontal lobe, may also give rise to apraxic disorders.

MOOD AND AFFECT

Mood and affect are two components of the psychologic profile of the patient. *Mood* refers to feelings and emotions evoked by situations, events, and other occurrences that characterize daily living. *Emotions* can be viewed as experiences of feelings associated with wants and needs that are met or unmet. Emotions are extremely varied and represent experiences known only to the patient. *Affect* refers to somatic and autonomic behaviors that are used to convey a mood or an emotion. These behaviors, like the feelings they reflect, can vary greatly and should be viewed in light of the patient's individual circumstances. When evaluating mood and affect, it is important to note whether you think the patient's behavior (affect) is consistent with what you believe to be the patient's emotional state and whether these seem to be appropriate or inappropriate in the context of the present circumstances.

THOUGHT CONTENT

Thought content refers to fullness and organization of the patient's thinking, as reflected in conversation and behavior. In neurologically intact individuals, thought content should be coherent and organized. Paranoia is an example of disordered thought content.

SUMMARY

The ability of the novice clinician to evaluate mental status accurately and reliably is likely to be somewhat limited at first. Experience and thoughtful review of the techniques used and their results will bring about a refinement and improvement in this important clinical skill.

The various tests of mental status described earlier are relatively simple in design and easily used in the office or at the bedside. Properly performed and interpreted, they should provide the examiner with a reliable assessment of mental status. More sensitive and descriptive methods of testing are available, however, particularly in the areas of language ability, memory and recall, and higher cortical function. Many of these tests have been developed by psychologists, speech pathologists, and other highly trained healthcare professionals. Individuals with these important skills should be sought out and consulted when disease conditions and treatment goals require a more thorough or sensitive evaluation of a patient's mental status.

4

CRANIAL NERVES

The cranial nerves are peripheral nerves that transmit impulses to and from the central nervous system. Cranial nerves, like spinal nerves, are composed of axons that subserve a variety of sensory, motor, and reflex functions. Some cranial nerves are afferent in function and others are exclusively efferent, but the majority are mixed, carrying information both to and from the brain.

The techniques for evaluating cranial nerve function are not particularly complicated if the examiner keeps in mind the functional components of each cranial nerve. Sensory deficits are present when afferent fibers are involved, and motor impairments are seen when efferent fibers are damaged. Reflexes involving cranial nerves can be affected by lesions that damage either afferent or efferent axons. Understanding of the basis for particular tests of cranial nerve function requires familiarity with the functional components of individual cranial nerves (Table 4). A working knowledge of the functional components of the cranial nerves is also necessary for the proper interpretation of signs and symptoms associated with cranial nerve lesions. Think of the process of testing cranial nerve function as an exercise in applied anatomy. Working from this perspective makes cranial nerve testing a logical and relatively uncomplicated process.

Table 4 is not exhaustive with regard to cranial nerve function; it merely indicates the functions that are clinically significant and that should be tested as part of the routine neurologic examination. In the following sections, each cranial nerve is considered individually, including:

- A brief description of pertinent anatomy, focusing on the location of cell bodies, the course of nerve fibers, and the target structure innervated

TABLE 4 *Functional Components of the Cranial Nerves*

Number	Name	Components	Function
I	Olfactory	Afferent	Olfaction (smell)
II	Optic	Afferent	Vision
III	Oculomotor	Efferent	
		Somatic	Elevates eyelid
			Turns eye up, down, in
		Visceral	Constricts pupil
			Accommodates lens
IV	Trochlear	Efferent (somatic)	Turns the adducted eye down and causes intorsion of eye
V	Trigeminal	Mixed	
		Afferent	Sensation from face
			Sensation from cornea
			Sensation from anterior tongue
		Efferent	Muscles of mastication
			Dampens sound (tensor tympani)
VI	Abducens	Efferent (somatic)	Turns eye out
VII	Facial	Mixed	
		Afferent	Taste from anterior tongue
		Efferent (somatic)	Muscles of facial expression
			Dampens sound (stapedius)
		Efferent (visceral)	Tearing (lacrimal gland)
			Salivation (submandibular and sublingual glands)
VIII	Vestibulocochlear	Afferent	Balance (semicircular canals, utricle, saccule)
			Hearing (organ of Corti)
IX	Glossopharyngeal	Mixed	
		Afferent	Taste from posterior tongue
			Sensation from posterior tongue
			Sensation from oropharynx
		Efferent	Salivation (parotid gland)
X	Vagus	Mixed	
		Afferent	Thoracic and abdominal viscera
		Efferent	Muscles of larynx and pharynx
			Decreases heart rate
			Increases GI motility
XI	Spinal accessory	Efferent	Head movements (sternocleidomastoid and trapezius)
XII	Hypoglossal	Efferent	Tongue movements and shape

GI = gastrointestinal.

- Simple procedures for testing functions associated with each cranial nerve
- A description of normal findings on these tests
- A brief description of some commonly encountered abnormal findings
- Methods for documenting both normal and abnormal observations

Proper testing technique is essential if the examiner expects a reliable assessment of cranial nerve function. An accurate and reliable interpretation of the results is possible only if the tests are performed properly. No less important is the ability to document and record clinical findings in a way that is meaningful and useful to others who may need the information. It is both embarrassing and troublesome if you have skillfully performed and correctly interpreted the findings of the neurologic examination but have failed to record and document your findings fully and accurately. A single foray into the legal system involving depositions and court appearances is always sufficient to bring home the necessity of being thorough, complete, precise, and clear in documentation.

OLFACTORY NERVE (I)

Functional Anatomy

The olfactory nerves are actually short nerve fibers that originate from bipolar neurons located in the mucous membrane in the roof of the nasal cavity. The axons collect into small fila, which course upward through the cribriform plate of the ethmoid bone to make synaptic contact with neurons in the olfactory bulb. The peripheral processes of these bipolar olfactory neurons are associated with chemoreceptive endings located in the olfactory epithelium. Axons of neurons located in the olfactory bulb constitute the olfactory tract, a distinct bundle of fibers that lies on the ventral surface of the frontal lobe in the olfactory sulcus. The axons of the olfactory tract terminate, among other places, in the medial temporal lobe, septal area, and hypothalamus, regions of the brain that are important in olfactory discrimination and the regulation of autonomic and emotional reactions to olfactory stimuli.

Clinical Examinations

Olfactory nerve function is tested by presenting non-noxious odorants such as coffee, soap, tobacco, or orange separately to each nostril. These substances can be stored in small, airtight vials for use when needed.

Each nostril should be visually inspected for obstructions that might impair airflow to the region of the olfactory epithelium. The patient should be instructed to occlude one nostril with a finger and asked if he or she smells something when the odorant is placed beneath the unoccluded nostril. It is helpful, although not necessary, for the patient to be able to identify the odorant. Failure to correctly identify an odorant might reflect lack of previous exposure to a particular odorant rather than an inability to detect olfactory stimuli. For this reason, common odorants should always be used.

Occasionally, it might be necessary to use sugar or some other substance that does not have an odor if there is reason to suspect that a patient may be engaging in confabulatory behavior. Do not use substances such as ammonia or other volatile, pungent chemicals because these produce reactions and reflex responses mediated by the trigeminal nerve. Nerve fibers in the nasal cavity associated with the trigeminal nerve are involved in signaling injury from chemical or mechanical causes rather than in detecting olfactory stimuli.

If the patient's sense of smell is intact, it should be so noted. Inability to detect odorants is referred to as *anosmia*. If anosmia is present, note whether it is bilateral or unilateral. The inability to recognize an odorant is referred to as *olfactory agnosia*.

OPTIC NERVE (II)

Functional Anatomy

The visual pathway begins in the retina and ends in the cortex of the occipital lobe, in and on either side of the calcarine sulcus. The nerve cell bodies and axons that compose the visual pathway are highly organized over their entire extent and terminate in a retinotopic fashion in the primary visual cortex (Brodmann's area 17). Figure 2 illustrates the major neural components of the visual pathway.

The functional integrity of the visual pathway is determined by testing visual acuity (central vision) and visual fields (peripheral vision). Certain components of the visual pathway are also important in regulating the size of the pupil (light reflexes) and adjusting the shape of the lens for near and far vision (accommodation reflex). Tests for these two functions are considered later in this section, together with the anatomic structures required for their normal function.

Clinical Examinations

Before performing any tests of visual function, it is important to inspect the eyes and eyelids for any asymmetries or abnormalities that might suggest a particular lesion or disease or that might lead the examiner to anticipate a particular response in subsequent testing. Inspection of the globes should include an assessment of their size and location within the orbit; their resting position relative to the line of sight (visual axis); pupillary size and shape; the condition of the iris, cornea, and retina; and the presence or absence of opacities of the lens.

The palpebral fissures should be inspected with regard to their size and the position of the lids relative to the iris and the pupil. Special attention should be directed to the position and symmetry of the upper eye-

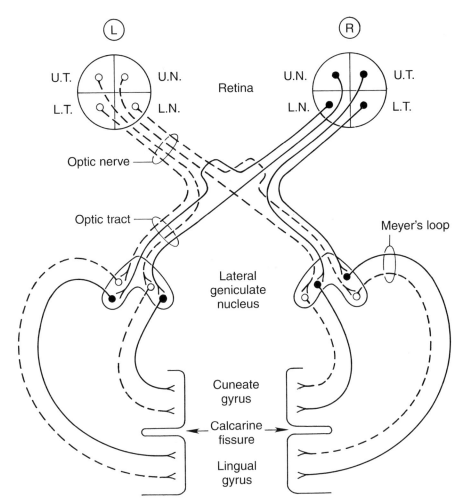

FIGURE 2. The visual pathway. U.N. = upper nasal quadrant, L.N. = lower nasal quadrant, U.T. = upper temporal quadrant, L.T. = lower temporal quadrant.

lids. *Ptosis* is a condition in which the upper eyelid droops, reducing the height of the palpebral fissure. In the resting position, with the eyes directed forward, the lower eyelid margin should be at the lower border of the iris or covering only a very small portion of the lower part of the iris. The upper eyelid margin should cover the upper part of the iris without encroaching on the pupil. The height of the palpebral fissure varies somewhat in the normal population, but should be equal bilaterally in a particular individual. It can be measured easily with a small pocket ruler, using the center of the pupil as a convenient reference point. Differences in the height of the palpebral fissures should be documented quantitatively; they usually result from injuries or disease conditions that affect the nerves innervating the muscles of the upper lid.

The levator palpebrae superioris, a skeletal muscle of the upper eyelid, is the major muscle involved in keeping the eye open. It is innervated by the oculomotor nerve. The upper eyelid also contains smooth muscle fibers (Müller's muscle) located in the tarsal plate. The smooth muscle fibers of the upper eyelid are innervated by sympathetic nerve fibers originating from postganglionic sympathetic neurons located in the ipsilateral superior cervical ganglion. Damage to either the oculomotor nerve or the sympathetic fibers innervating Müller's muscle can produce drooping of the upper eyelid. Lesions of the oculomotor nerve produce a constellation of findings that includes ptosis that does not resolve with upward gaze, corectasia (dilated pupil), exotropia (lateral deviation), and hypotropia (downward deviation) of the eye in the position of primary gaze, cycloplegia (inability to accommodate the lens for near vision), and diplopia (double vision) with lateral gaze to the contralateral side. Lesions that damage the sympathetic innervation to Müller's muscle, on the other hand, produce ptosis that disappears with upward gaze, together with miosis (constricted pupil), anhidrosis (absence of sweating), and hyperemia (redness) on the ipsilateral side of the face. The clinical condition resulting from injuries or lesions involving the sympathetic innervation of structures in the head is referred to as *Horner's syndrome.*

The globes should be equal in size, shape, and location within the orbit. *Proptosis* (exophthalmos) is a condition in which the globes appear to be bulging out of the orbits. The size and position of the globes can easily be determined with the patient seated in a chair and the examiner standing behind the patient looking down from above. An ophthalmometer can be used if needed to obtain a more precise, quantitative measure of the position of each globe in the orbit.

Ocular alignment can be determined in a number of ways. A simple method that is appropriate for screening at this point in the neurologic examination is the *corneal light reflection test* (corneal light reflex). This test is performed in a darkened room with the patient and examiner sitting face to face. The patient is instructed to focus on some distant object in line with the top of the examiner's head. The examiner then places a penlight in the midline beneath his or her own chin and aims the light beam at the patient's chin or nose. The reflection of a point of light should be seen in each pupil. If ocular alignment is normal, the points of light should be seen slightly inferior and medial to the center of the pupil. If an eye is deviated in a particular direction, the corneal light reflection will be displaced in the opposite direction. The mechanical basis for the

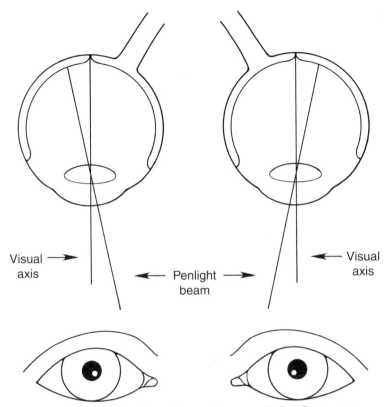

FIGURE 3. The mechanical basis of the corneal light reflection test.

corneal light reflex is illustrated in Figure 3. Lesions resulting in ocular malalignment will be discussed later, when we consider tests of extraocular muscle function, but this simple screening test can be used to identify gross abnormalities of ocular alignment that might influence the results of tests of visual acuity and visual fields.

Pupillary size and shape should be examined by visual inspection. The pupils should be equal in size and shape, measuring approximately 3 mm in diameter in ambient light and 5 mm in dim light, the level of light that will be required for testing the light reflexes. Resting pupil size in the normal population decreases slightly with age. In addition, a slight inequality in pupil size (anisocoria) is not uncommon. Between 15 and 30 percent of normal individuals demonstrate an inequality of 0.4 mm or greater. *Corectasia* and *mydriasis* are terms used to refer to a pupil that is dilated or larger than normal. A *miotic* pupil is one that is constricted or smaller than normal.

The cornea and lens should also be examined with the naked eye and with the ophthalmoscope. Both should be clear and free of opacities. Both retinas should also be examined, with specific reference to the appearance of the fovea centralis, the optic disk or cup, and the vessels that emerge from the optic disk.

Funduscopic Examination

Examination of the internal structures of the eye with an ophthalmoscope is an important part of the neurologic examination. Students and inexperienced clinicians are encouraged to examine the fundi in all patients whether or not there are complaints of visual problems. Familiarity with the normal appearance of structures in the eye is a necessary prerequisite for being able to recognize abnormality when it is present.

The examination should be performed in a darkened room to promote dilatation of the pupil. The routine use of mydriatic agents is neither necessary nor encouraged. The patient should be instructed to keep both eyes open and focus on some distant point in the room. The examiner should use his or her right eye to examine the patient's right eye and the left eye to examine the patient's left eye. The examiner also needs to learn to use the ophthalmoscope with either hand. Sometimes the examiner needs to hold the patient's lid up with his or her free hand.

Structures of interest in the funduscopic examination include the optic disk and cup, retinal vessels, and macula. The optic disk is circular in form, approximately 1.5 mm in diameter, and pale pink in color. The margins of the disk should be clear and distinct, with the temporal margin slightly sharper than the nasal edge. The nasal side of the disk may be slightly pinker than the temporal side, owing to the greater density of blood vessels. The optic cup, located centrally within the disk, is a well-defined depression in the optic nerve head and is paler than the more peripheral parts of the disk. The normal optic cup should be no more than 40 percent of the size of the optic disk.

Retinal vessels emerge from the optic cup and branch mainly in superior and inferior directions before further dividing. Retinal arteries and veins are paired and cross the disk margins to supply the retina. Retinal arteries are two thirds the diameter of their corresponding veins and may appear slightly redder in color. Retinal veins may be seen to pulsate, but the absence of pulsations does not necessarily indicate pathology.

The macula is located two disk diameters to the temporal side of the optic disk. At the center of the macula is a small, pinpoint-sized white spot known as the *fovea centralis*. The fovea is the region of the retina of greatest visual acuity. The macula and the fovea should be free of retinal blood vessels.

In myopic individuals, the optic disks may be larger and paler than normal. In hypermetropic persons, the disks may be smaller and pinker. *Papilledema*, swelling of the optic nerve head, can be seen in patients with increased intracranial pressure or optic neuritis. Characteristic features of papilledema include disks that are pinker than normal, enlarged veins that do not pulsate, blurring of the disk margins especially on the nasal side, vessels that appear elevated as they cross the disk margins, and sometimes hemorrhages and exudates near the disk edge.

The reader is referred to standard texts of ophthalmology for further details regarding the normal appearance of retinal structures and characteristics of specific disease processes that may be encountered in the routine neurologic examination.

Visual Acuity

Visual acuity tests are designed to assess the integrity and function of those parts of the visual pathway required for fine visual discrimination, generally considered to be 20 degrees radially from the point of fixation. The macular region of the retina and the occipital poles are of particular importance in this regard. The macula lutea, which contains the fovea centralis, is in direct line with the visual axis. This region of the retina is characterized by a high concentration of cones and the relative absence of other cellular layers of the retina through which light must pass. The macular region of the retina is the region of highest visual acuity and is important in functions requiring a high degree of visual discrimination, such as reading.

Visual acuity is tested in each eye separately. If the patient wears glasses or contact lenses to correct for refraction errors, they should be worn during testing. The environment in which the tests are conducted should be well lit, comfortable for the patient, and free of distracting stimuli. The patient is first instructed to cover one eye with the palm of the hand. With the uncovered eye, the patient is asked to read letters or numbers printed on standard charts used for this purpose. Distant vision can be assessed in the clinic or examiner's office with the aid of a Snellen chart, a wall-mounted chart placed at a distance of 20 ft from the patient. Alternatively, a more convenient pocket-sized card (Rosenbaum Pocket Vision Screener) may be used. The pocket-sized card is held 14 inches from the eye and contains numbers, letters, and other symbols of differing sizes that the patient is asked to identify. Both testing instruments indicate distance equivalents that are used in recording degree of visual acuity. Normal visual acuity is recorded as 20/20, which means that the patient can distinguish numbers or letters at 20 ft that an individual with normal vision (standard vision) can distinguish at 20 ft. A patient with standard vision is referred to as *emmetropic*. If, however, the patient can distinguish only at 20 ft what the normal eye can distinguish at 100 ft, visual acuity would be recorded as 20/100 for that eye. The denominator in the record refers to the distance at which an individual with normal visual acuity can distinguish the numbers or letters on the test instrument. *Myopia* (nearsightedness) refers to an acuity deficit in which distant vision is impaired while near vision is normal. Images from distant objects are focused in front of the retina and thus are out of focus to the patient. Myopia can occur with aging and is usually the result of processes that increase the size (anteroposterior diameter) of the eye. *Hyperopia* (farsightedness) refers to a condition in which near images are focused behind the retina; distance vision is normal while near vision may be blurred. If near vision is blurred, it is either because the degree of hyperopia is severe or because the patient also suffers from *presbyopia*, a condition characterized by a decreased ability of the lens to accommodate (become more round) for near vision. Presbyopia may develop with increasing age.

Visual Fields

Visual fields should always be examined, because patients may be unaware of subtle, small, or slowly developing visual field defects. Moreover, unexpected findings frequently have a way of gaining importance, particularly when considered in the context of specific patient complaints or in conjunction with other historical or examination data.

The normal visual fields are not circular, but rather somewhat irregular in shape, extending 60 degrees above, 60 degrees medial, 75 degrees below, and 100 degrees lateral from the visual axis in primary gaze. With both eyes open, an appreciable overlap is seen between the medial or nasal visual fields of both eyes.

A variety of procedures can be used to assess visual fields, depending on the degree of precision required. The simplest method for evaluating visual fields is by *confrontation tests*. These tests are particularly useful for examinations performed at the bedside or in other clinical settings where specialized equipment is not available. The room should be well lit and free from distractions that might otherwise capture the attention of the patient. The examiner and patient should be comfortably situated face to face, separated by no more than 50 to 60 cm. The patient should be instructed to cover one eye and look directly at the examiner's nose with the uncovered eye. If the left eye of the patient is to be tested first, the examiner's own left eye should be closed so that the examiner's open right eye is looking directly at the patient's open left eye. The examiner thereby can use his or her own visual field as a comparison or control in the test.

To perform the test, the examiner presents a static visual stimulus — one, two, or three fingers — to each of the four diagonal visual quadrants. The patient is asked to indicate how many fingers are seen on each presentation without shifting focus from the examiner's nose. Multiple presentations should be made in each visual quadrant. If the patient is unable to report the number of fingers presented to a particular visual field accurately, a field defect is suspected. More sophisticated testing requiring specialized equipment will be needed if a more precise mapping of the extent of the field defect is desired. After one eye is tested and the examiner is satisfied with the findings, the other eye should be tested using the same procedure. Field defects should be documented and described in the patient's chart.

Confrontation testing is a reliable method of testing visual fields if care is taken to perform the test properly and, of course, if the examiner's own visual fields are normal. If questionable findings are present or if field defects are uncovered, more sensitive testing may be required. A more accurate assessment of the periphery of the visual field can be obtained by means of *perimeter testing. Tangent screen testing* is useful for examining the more central portions of each visual field. Each of these tests requires specialized equipment that may not be generally available in the clinic or at the bedside. The results of these types of tests can be of great importance in certain situations, however, and the tests should be performed without hesitation if a more complete assessment of the visual fields is needed.

Visual field defects are named to reflect the direction or directions from which the patient cannot see. For example, a patient with a defect involving only the right eye who is unable to see things to the left would be reported to have a left hemianopsia involving the right eye. If the patient is unable to see things to the left with either eye, the condition is referred to as a left homonymous hemianopsia. *Homonymous* refers to the fact that defects in the same direction are present in the visual fields of both eyes. Homonymous defects are seen in patients with lesions involving components of the visual pathway on one side, behind the level of the optic chiasm.

Visual field defects can be restricted to a single quarter, or quadrant, of the visual field. Such defects are referred to as *quadrantanopsias* and are named to reflect the quadrant of the visual field from which the patient is unable to see. For example, a patient with a defect involving only the left eye who is unable to see objects below and to the right would be reported to have an inferior nasal quadrantanopsia of the left eye. If the patient is unable to see objects below and to the right with either eye, the condition would be referred to as right inferior homonymous quadrantanopsia. Lesions involving the white matter in the middle part of the temporal lobe can damage part of the optic radiations extending from the lateral geniculate nucleus to the primary visual cortex in the occipital lobe (Meyer's loop). These axons subserve the lower temporal retinal quadrant of the ipsilateral eye and the lower nasal retinal quadrant of the contralateral eye. Such a lesion on the right side, for example, would result in a *left superior* homonymous quadrantanopsia. In general, visual field defects restricted to one eye suggest prechiasmatic disease processes, whereas defects identified in both eyes, frequently homonymous in character, indicate postchiasmal lesions. Isolated quadrantanopsias restricted to the superior temporal visual field of one or both eyes may suggest lesions involving the white matter in the contralateral temporal lobe. To clarify these concepts, review Figure 2, and keep in mind that the lens inverts and reverses images before they reach the retina.

Other types of visual field defects are encountered from time to time. Complete blindness in one eye is referred to as *anopsia* (anopia) and may indicate significant damage or complete destruction of the optic nerve. Occasionally, pituitary tumors damage axons crossing the midline in the optic chiasm. Because these axons originate from ganglion cells located in the nasal retinal quadrants of each eye, the resulting visual field defect would be referred to as a *bitemporal* (heteronymous) *hemianopsia*. The degree to which this finding is observed reflects the degree to which the fibers crossing in the optic chiasm are damaged.

Lesions or changes involving the retina or media of the eye may produce small, localized visual field defects that the patient may see as small, dark spots. Such localized defects are referred to as *positive scotomas*. Conversely, lesions involving the optic nerve head or optic nerve can produce a slightly different type of visual field defect, characterized by an arc of diminished visual acuity (relative scotomas) or by an apparent blank space in the visual world (absolute or negative scotomas). These latter scotomas may vary in size and location and sometimes go unnoticed by the patient. For this reason, it is important to evaluate the patient's visual fields even when there is no complaint of visual disturbances.

Visual Reflexes

Normal vision requires more than simply a nerve pathway for transmitting impulses from the retina to the primary visual cortex. Because light conditions vary from place to place and from time to time, a mechanism is needed to regulate the amount of light that reaches the retina. Such regulation is achieved by reflex mechanisms that control the size of the pupil.

Similarly, because objects of interest can be located both near and far from the individual, a mechanism is needed to control the relative position of the eyes so that the image of the object of interest always falls on the macular portions of both retinas. In these situations, it is also desirable to be able to adjust the focal length of the optical system so that the object is always clearly in focus, regardless of its distance from the individual. Mechanisms to mediate these related functions do exist and involve both the extraocular muscles and the intrinsic smooth muscles of the eye. We now consider techniques for evaluating the integrity of these two reflex mechanisms related to vision.

The Light Reflexes

The iris contains smooth muscles oriented radially and circularly around the pupil. The radially oriented smooth muscles cause the pupil to dilate and are under the control of the sympathetic division of the autonomic nervous system. The dilator muscles are innervated by neurons located in the superior cervical ganglion, which are adrenergic in nature. The circularly oriented smooth muscles cause constriction of the pupil and are under the control of the parasympathetic division of the autonomic nervous system. These muscles are innervated by neurons located in the ciliary ganglion and are cholinergic in nature. The ciliary ganglion is innervated by axons carried in the oculomotor nerve; these axons originate from nerve cell bodies located in the Edinger-Westphal nucleus.

Constriction is the normal response of the pupil to an increase in light intensity, whereas dilatation of the pupil normally occurs in response to a reduction in light intensity. The afferent limb of the light reflex is made up of the axons of ganglion cells of the retina, which compose the optic nerves, chiasm, and optic tracts. Collateral branches of these axons terminate in the pretectal area, which in turn transmits nerve impulses to lower motor neurons, which influence the pupillary constrictors. The efferent limb of the reflex consists of the axons of cells located in the Edinger-Westphal nucleus, which enter the orbit as part of the oculomotor nerve, and the axons of neurons found in the ciliary ganglion, which compose the short ciliary nerves. Figure 4 illustrates the neural pathways and structures involved in the light reflexes.

The light reflexes must be tested in a dimly lit room to properly elicit and visualize the normal pupillary responses. The patient is instructed to look straight ahead and to focus on some point in the distance (to avoid constriction of the pupil that accompanies convergence). The examiner then brings the bright light of a penlight from the side of the patient's head into one eye. The examiner may place the edge of one hand against the patient's nose and forehead to prevent light from reaching the patient's other eye, which should remain open during the test. Pupillary reactions in both eyes should be examined and duly recorded. Normally, the pupils of both eyes should promptly constrict. The pupillary constriction observed in the illuminated eye is referred to as the *direct light reflex*, and the response in the nonilluminated eye is referred to as the *indirect, consensual*, or *crossed-light reflex*. *Iridoplegia* is a term used to describe a condition in which the pupil does not react to light stimulation. An *amau-*

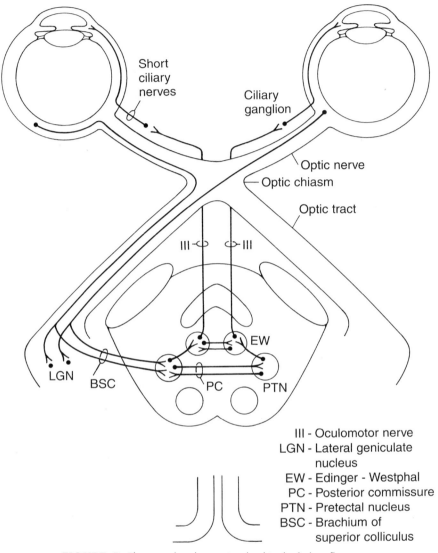

FIGURE 4. The neural pathways involved in the light reflexes.

rotic pupil is one that does not constrict in response to light; it is seen in a patient whose retina or optic nerve has been completely destroyed.

A useful test of pupillary function is the *swinging flashlight test*. In this test, the patient is asked to focus on a distant object in a darkened room. Darkening the examining room not only causes dilatation of the patient's pupils, which is necessary if responses to light stimuli are to be seen, but also dilates the pupils of the examiner so that he or she will be better able to observe the patient's pupillary responses. The examiner then shines a penlight alternately into one eye and then the other, each time carefully observing the pupillary response in both eyes. The rate at which the light is moved from eye to eye may vary but should be approximately 1 cycle per second. The normal response is constriction of both pupils when the light is directed into each eye, with a slight dilatation bilaterally as the light moves across the bridge of the nose. The light-stimulated pupil constricts as a result of the direct light reflex, while the nonstimulated pupil constricts as a result of the indirect light reflex.

A patient with damage to the optic nerve, but without loss of visual acuity, may demonstrate a paradoxic pupillary response. When light enters the normal eye, both pupils constrict, the stimulated (normal) eye demonstrating a direct light reflex and the nonstimulated (abnormal) eye demonstrating an indirect or consensual light reflex. When the light is shifted to the abnormal eye, both pupils dilate because of a relative reduction in the intensity of light that is available to provoke the direct and indirect light reflexes. If the examiner again shifts the light to the normal eye, both pupils constrict promptly. This observation, which indicates damage to the optic nerve on the side at which dilatation occurred in response to light stimulation, is referred to as an *afferent pupillary deficit* (Marcus Gunn pupil).

In a patient with an isolated oculomotor nerve lesion, the pupil in that eye will remain dilated (mydriatic) regardless of which eye is stimulated. The pupil demonstrates neither a direct nor an indirect light reflex. The pupil in the normal eye will constrict when the light is shone into either eye.

Both the direct and indirect light reflexes should be evaluated in both eyes. The light reflexes are documented as being present, absent, or diminished. Documentation of light reflex abnormalities should always make clear which reflexes are abnormal and whether one or both eyes are involved. The most common mistake made in testing the light reflexes is the use of a light source that is not sufficiently bright to elicit a normal response. The next most common mistake is failure to record test results in the patient's chart.

Accommodation Reflex

The accommodation reflex is a normal response that comes into play when there is a need to view an object at near distances (20 cm or less). The intent of this automatic response is to adjust the position of the globes so that the image of the object being viewed falls on the fovea of both eyes and to adjust the shape of the lens to maintain sharp focus at near distances.

The afferent limb of the accommodation reflex includes the retina, optic nerves, chiasm, tracts and radiations, and the visual cortex. The efferent limb involves two components: lower motor neurons of the oculomotor nucleus, which innervate the medial rectus muscle, and autonomic (parasympathetic) neurons, which control the pupillary constrictor and ciliary muscles. The medial rectus acts to adduct the eyes. The pupillary constrictor muscle is responsible for reducing the diameter of the pupil, whereas the ciliary muscle is responsible for reducing tension on the lens, thereby permitting the lens to assume a slightly rounder, more convex shape. The axons to all three muscle groups involved in the accommodation reflex emerge from the rostral midbrain and are carried into the orbit as part of the oculomotor nerve. Figure 5 illustrates the neural pathways and structures involved in the accommodation reflex.

The reflex is tested by asking the patient to focus both eyes on the examiner's finger as it is slowly advanced toward the patient's nose from a distance of approximately 60 cm (2 ft). Alternatively, the examiner can place one finger approximately 8 cm in front of the patient's nose and ask the patient to shift his or her focus of vision back and forth between the examiner's finger and an object in line with the finger, but at some significant distance away. The examiner should carefully observe the patient's eyes for two responses: convergence (ocular adduction) and constriction of the pupil. A third component of the accommodation reflex, a change in the shape of the lens to a more convex form, is not visible to the examiner but can be inferred to have occurred if the patient reports that the finger remained in focus as it was moved toward the nose or as vision is shifted to the finger at close range. Accommodation is considered to be impaired if one or both eyes do not converge or the pupils do not constrict. Rarely, however, one response may be present in the absence of the other. When documenting an impairment of the accommodation reflex, it is important to note the side of impairment, if unilateral, and which component of the reflex is abnormal.

OCULAR MOTOR NERVES

The oculomotor, trochlear, and abducens nerves are involved in a variety of ocular motor functions. All three nerves provide motor innervation to the extraocular muscles. In addition, the oculomotor nerve innervates the elevator of the upper eyelid (levator palpebrae superioris) and regulates pupil size and lens shape. In clinical practice, the voluntary and reflex functions mediated by these cranial nerves are generally tested together. Tests of ocular motor function are exercises in applied anatomy, easily understood and performed if the examiner keeps in mind simple anatomic relationships peculiar to the eye and each cranial nerve. Following is a brief review of these important anatomic relationships.

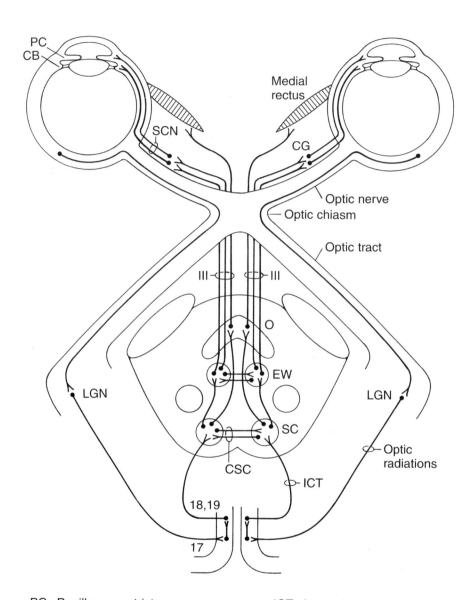

PC - Pupillary constrictor
CB - Ciliary body
SCN - Short ciliary nerves
O - Oculomotor nucleus (nucleus perlia)
III - Oculomotor nerve
EW - Edinger - Westphal
SC - Superior colliculus

ICT - Internal corticotectal tract
CSC - Commissure of
      superior colliculus
CG - Ciliary ganglion
17 - Occipital lobe (area 17)
18,19 - Occipital lobe (area 18, 19)
LGN - Lateral geniculate nucleus

FIGURE 5. The neural pathways involved in the accommodation reflex.

Functional Anatomy

Movements of the globe are produced by six extraocular muscles. A clear understanding of the origin, insertion, and action of each extraocular muscle is absolutely essential if the examiner hopes to understand the rationale behind particular test maneuvers and their interpretation. Such knowledge is equally necessary for an understanding of the signs and symptoms associated with ocular motor dysfunction. Figure 6 illustrates the ocular attachments of the extraocular muscles. Note that in the position of primary gaze (Fig. 6A), the muscle fibers of the superior oblique and inferior oblique muscles lie largely medial to a vertical axis through the globe. The muscle fibers of the superior and inferior rectus muscles also lie medial to the vertical axis. In the position of primary gaze, the angle formed by the visual axis and the fibers of the superior and inferior rectus muscles is approximately 21 degrees, and the angle formed by the visual axis and the fibers of the superior and inferior oblique muscles is roughly 51 degrees. This observation suggests that, in this position, the major action of the superior rectus muscle would be to elevate the globe, whereas the inferior rectus muscle would act to depress it; the superior oblique muscle would cause intorsion of the eye, and the inferior oblique muscle would cause extorsion of it. In point of fact, in the position of primary gaze all six muscles are active to a greater or lesser degree. The actions of the medial and lateral rectus muscles effectively offset one another so that the eye is neither adducted nor abducted. The actions of the superior and inferior rectus muscles are balanced so that the eye is neither elevated nor depressed, and the actions of the superior and inferior oblique muscles are balanced so that the eye undergoes neither intorsion nor extorsion when in the position of primary gaze.

Movements of the eye occur as a result of the coordinated contraction and relaxation of opposing muscle pairs. The clinical significance of these anatomic details, particularly the fact that muscles are paired to pull the eye in equal and opposite directions, will become obvious when we consider the signs and symptoms produced by nerve injuries and other conditions that upset this delicate balance.

The particular action of each muscle on the globe is also influenced by the position of the globe within the orbit. When the eye is adducted, as for reading or viewing objects at close distances, the axis of ocular rotation relative to the pull of certain muscles changes. The superior oblique muscle becomes a depressor of the eye, whereas the inferior oblique muscle acts to elevate it. The superior and inferior rectus muscles assume a slight role in ocular intorsion and extorsion respectively. The altered mechanical relationships that are seen when the eye is adducted are illustrated in Figure 6B.

When the eye is abducted, as depicted in Figure 6B, the superior and

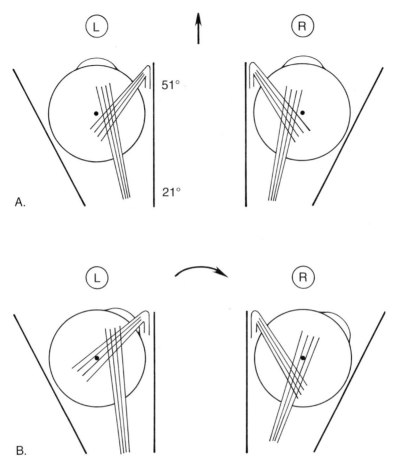

FIGURE 6. The relationship of the tendons and insertions of four extraocular muscles to a vertical axis through the eye. *A* illustrates these relationships when the eyes are in the position of primary gaze. *B* illustrates these relationships when the eyes are turned to the right. Note that the movements produced by a particular muscle are influenced by the position of the eye.

inferior rectus muscles become the primary elevators and depressors of the eye; contraction of the superior and inferior oblique muscles results in intorsion and extorsion of the eye respectively.

Obviously, a grasp of these simple but important anatomic relationships is essential to an understanding of tests of extraocular function; these relationships form the basis of judgments regarding the nature of specific ocular motor deficits. Readers who feel unsure should review them again so that they can be applied without hesitation in the clinical setting.

The motor innervation of each extraocular muscle is indicated in Table 5. In addition to the extraocular muscles listed in the table, the oculomotor nerve also innervates the levator palpebrae superioris, the constrictor of the pupil, and the ciliary muscle of the eye, which regulates the shape of the lens.

Several other clinically significant facts about the innervation of the extraocular muscles should be mentioned before considering tests of ocular motor function. The abducens nucleus innervates the ipsilateral rectus muscle, whereas the trochlear nucleus provides motor innervation to the contralateral superior oblique muscle. The crossing of the trochlear nerve fibers occurs intra-axially, within the superior medullary velum, before the axons emerge from the dorsal surface of the brainstem immediately caudal to the inferior colliculus. The nuclear origin of fibers in the oculomotor nerve is a bit more complicated. Nerve fibers innervating the medial rectus, inferior rectus, and inferior oblique muscles originate from subnuclei of the oculomotor nuclear complex on the ipsilateral side, whereas fibers destined for the superior rectus muscle originate from neurons in the contralateral oculomotor nucleus. The crossing of these latter fibers occurs within the oculomotor nuclear complex, immediately beneath the central gray matter at the level of the superior colliculus. The levator palpebrae superioris is bilaterally innervated by neurons in the oculomotor nucleus of both sides. The crossing of the crossed component also occurs within the oculomotor nuclear complex, immediately ventral to the central gray matter. The innervation of the pupillary constrictor muscle and the ciliary muscle is derived from neurons in the ipsilateral ciliary ganglion, which itself is innervated by oculomotor nerve fibers originating from neurons located on the ipsilateral side in the Edinger-Westphal nucleus (see Fig. 5).

General Considerations

The examination of ocular motor function should always begin with the examiner asking the patient about any problems he or she may be having with regard to vision. Complaints of double vision (diplopia), blurring of

TABLE 5   *Cranial Nerve Innervation of the Extraocular Muscles*

	Cranial Nerve	Muscle Innervated
	III	Superior rectus
		Inferior rectus
		Medial rectus
		Inferior oblique
	IV	Superior oblique
	VI	Lateral rectus

vision at near or far distances, differences in perceived light intensity between the two eyes, blind spots (scotomas), or pain with eye movements should alert the examiner to the existence of a specific problem and serve to focus attention on particular aspects of the ocular motor examination. Visual inspection of the eyelids and palpebral fissures, the pupils, and the position of the eyes in primary gaze is an important part of the evaluation at this time, yielding valuable information about the functional integrity of cranial nerves III, IV, and VI. Although the eyelids and pupils have already been observed while evaluating visual acuity and visual fields, it is worthwhile to look at them again in the context of evaluating ocular motor function.

Ptosis can result from lesions involving the oculomotor nerve or the sympathetic innervation of Müller's muscle in the tarsal plate of the upper eyelid. Clinical findings useful in the differential diagnosis of ptosis were described in a previous section; becoming comfortable with this information is critical.

Pupillary function is evaluated by testing the light reflexes and accommodation reflex, as already discussed. The reader should practice these techniques frequently to acquire skill in their performance and experience in distinguishing normal from abnormal responses.

Clinical Examinations

Before performing particular tests of ocular motor function, it is important to observe the relative position of each eye within the orbit in primary gaze. The patient should be asked to look straight ahead and focus on some distant object in a well-lit room. Normally, the eyes are steady in the orbits and appear to be directed straight ahead. There should be no complaint of blurred vision or diplopia.

In some patients, the eyes do not appear to be looking straight ahead in a parallel manner. Malalignment of the visual axes, which is evident when the patient is free to look with both eyes and attempts to focus on a distant object, is referred to as *heterotropia*. Heterotropias are any manifest ocular deviations of the visual axis of an eye when the patient is given free central vision and is asked to fixate on some distant point. The term *strabismus* is sometimes used to refer to a misalignment of the visual axis. Heterotropias are named for the direction of deviation of the abnormal eye. Table 6 indicates terms used to refer to particular types of heterotropias. Some deviations are in the diagonal direction and must be described to indicate the direction of ocular deviation accurately.

Heterotropias can be congenital. In adults, they are most often acquired and result from weakness or paralysis involving one or more extraocular muscles in one eye. They may also be the result of conditions

TABLE 6 *Descriptive Characteristics of Manifest Ocular Deviations*

Name	Ocular Deviation
Exotropia	Eye turned outward (abducted)
Esotropia	Eye turned inward (adducted)
Hypertropia	Eye turned upward (supraducted)
Hypotropia	Eye turned downward (subducted)

that mechanically restrict the range of motion of the eye. Heterotropia may or may not be evident on primary gaze. If it is not apparent on primary gaze, it may become apparent when gaze is shifted in one direction or another. Subtle heterotropias may escape the notice of the examiner until they come to his or her attention in association with a complaint of diplopia. For these reasons, it is important to test ocular motor function carefully in all patients, regardless of whether they complain of diplopia or other visual disturbance.

A simple, objective test of ocular motor function is to ask the patient to hold his or her head still and look in specific directions while the examiner carefully observes the movement of the eyes. The directions of movement are specific and are based on the actions of particular extraocular muscles. Figure 7 illustrates the ocular movements the patient should perform and indicates the extraocular muscles that are involved in moving the eye into that position. The numbers represent a suggested order of movement. The room should be well lit and free from moving distractions within the patient's field of vision. Dysconjugate eye movements indicate heterotropia.

In an alternative and more sensitive subjective test, the examiner asks the patient to hold his or her head steady and follow a finger or penlight as it is moved into different positions in front of the patient. The examiner inquires carefully about the presence of double vision and notes the eye movements and positions that produce the greatest degree of diplopia.

Weakness or paralysis of one or more extraocular muscles results in heterotropia when the eyes are moved in the direction corresponding to the action of those muscles. For example, paralysis of the right lateral rectus muscle produces heterotropia (with diplopia) when the patient is asked to move his or her eyes laterally to the right. A finding of heterotropia during binocular testing should always be followed by monocular testing of each eye to firmly establish the abnormal functioning of the eye suspected to be at fault. Both the eye and the direction of movement deficit should be carefully documented. In the example just given, the

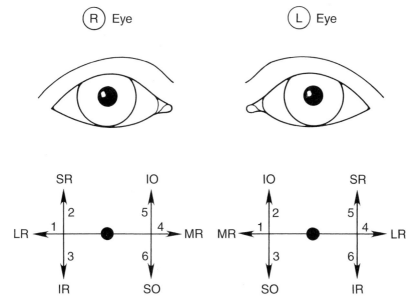

FIGURE 7. Movements produced by individual extraocular muscles. Numbers refer to a suggested order of voluntary or following movements intended to ensure complete assessment of ocular motor function. LR = lateral rectus, SR = superior rectus, IR = inferior rectus, MR = medial rectus, IO = inferior oblique, SO = superior oblique.

report should indicate that the right eye fails to abduct with right lateral gaze.

If the degree of ocular misalignment is the same regardless of the position of the eyes, the heterotropia is said to be *comitant*. Such comitant heterotropias are frequently congenital and may not be associated with diplopia, because the patient may have learned to suppress the visual input from one eye. If the degree of ocular misalignment changes with eye position, the heterotropia is said to be *noncomitant*. Noncomitant heterotropias are generally acquired and are the result of weak or paralyzed extraocular muscles. These heterotropias are typically associated with diplopia, which is maximal in the direction of pull of the weak or paralytic muscle.

Another test of ocular motor function is the *corneal light reflection test* (corneal light reflex), which was briefly described in a previous section. In performing this test to evaluate ocular motor function, the examiner places the penlight beneath his or her own chin and directs the beam at the patient's nose. The patient is asked to fixate on some point in the distance in line with the top of the examiner's head.

The examiner observes the reflection of the light beam on the patient's cornea, which in the normal individual should be slightly inferior and medial to the center of the pupil (see Fig. 3). With the patient fixating the gaze on a distant point as described, the examiner then turns the patient's head in the six directions indicated in Figure 7. In the normal individual, the eyes should not move and the corneal light reflections in each eye should remain fixed, slightly below and medial to the center of the pupil. In a patient with weak or paralyzed extraocular muscles, the light reflection will move in the opposite direction of the pull of the weak or paralyzed muscle. A patient with paralysis of the right lateral rectus muscle should demonstrate a lateral displacement of the light reflection in the right eye when the head is turned to the left. At this point, readers should think through these test maneuvers to be certain that they thoroughly understand why the light reflection moves on the cornea and the direction in which it will move in response to weakness or paralysis of a particular eye muscle.

Still another useful test of ocular motor function is the *red glass test.* A red glass is placed in front of one eye (by convention, the right eye), and the patient is asked to focus on a bright light source in the distance. The light source should be far enough away to avoid activating the accommodation response. The test permits the patient and the examiner to distinguish the image falling on each retina and to see double images more easily. The principles behind the red glass test are the same as for the corneal light reflex. The patient is asked to describe the amount of separation between the white and red light images as the eyes are moved in each of the six directions indicated in Figure 7, or as the examiner moves the patient's head into various positions.

Two simple rules can be applied when interpreting the findings of the red glass test. First, the degree of separation is greatest when the eyes are moved in the direction of pull of the weak or paralyzed muscle. Second, the more peripherally seen light image is always the "false" image and is seen by the eye with the weak or paralyzed muscle. The second rule assumes that the patient uses the nonparetic or normal eye to fixate during testing.

For example, let us assume that the red glass is in front of the right eye and the patient experiences diplopia with maximum separation of the red and white images while following the light stimulus into right lateral gaze. The conclusion to be drawn at this point is that the weak muscle is either the right lateral rectus muscle or the left medial rectus muscle. If the white image is displaced most peripherally in the field of vision, the weakness or paralysis must involve the left medial rectus muscle. The basis for this conclusion is that if the left eye is unable to follow the light stimulus as it is moved to the right, the light image will fall on the retina at some distance away from the macula, giving rise to the perception that the light source is located somewhere in the periphery. In this case, the white light will fall to the temporal side of the macula of the left eye, so the white image will appear to the right of the red image. If, on the other hand, the red image is located farther toward the periphery of the visual field, the weakness or paralysis must involve the lateral rectus muscle of the right eye because in this instance the right eye will be unable to follow the light, which will fall on the retina at some distance away from the macula. In this case, the red light will fall to the nasal side of the macula of the right eye, and the red image will appear to the right of the white image.

Another simple rule that might be helpful in interpreting the results of the red glass test is that a patient with an esotropia will have an uncrossed diplopia, whereas a patient with an exotropia will present with a crossed diplopia. The essence of this rule is that the diplopia described by a patient with an esotropia viewing with both eyes is characterized by the red image being to the right of the white image. Conversely, the diplopia reported by a patient with an exotropia will be characterized by the red image being to the left of the white image. A patient with an esotropia involving the right eye will see the red image to the right of the white image. A patient with an exotropia involving the right eye will perceive the red image to the left of the white image. Again, the reader should work through the logic and mechanics of these tests to become comfortable with the simple principles involved.

The *cover-uncover* (alternate uncover) *test* can also be used to assess ocular motor function. It is most useful in patients who do not demonstrate impairment on monocular or binocular ocular motor testing, in whom it helps to detect and distinguish latent ocular deviations (heterophorias) from manifest ocular malalignment conditions (heterotropias). *Heterophorias* are ocular deviations present only when central vision is occluded or when binocular vision is not permitted. *Heterotropias*, by contrast, are seen in patients whose central vision is not occluded and who are viewing with both eyes.

The cover-uncover test is performed in a well-lit room free of moving objects. The patient should be seated comfortably and asked to fixate vision on some distant object in the field of primary vision. The examiner then covers one of the patient's eyes and observes the response in the other eye. If the uncovered eye was fixating, it will not move. If the uncovered eye moves, the covered eye was fixating and the patient has a heterophoria. If the uncovered eye abducts, the patient has an esophoria involving that eye; if it adducts, the patient has an exophoria. Downward movement indicates a hyperphoria, and upward movement, a hypophoria.

In an alternative form of the cover-uncover test, the patient is asked to focus and maintain his or her vision on some distant point while the examiner moves the patient's head into each of the six positions indicated in Figure 7. In each position, the examiner blocks the vision of one eye and then the other while watching for movement of the eyes. Movement of the eye away from the point of fixation when vision is occluded, followed by a return of fixation when vision is restored, is indicative of heterophoria. Heterophorias are named by the direction of deviation that occurs under the occluded eye, using the same prefixes as used in naming heterotropias. For example, with the head turned to the left, if the right eye deviates medially when covered but moves laterally once again when uncovered, the condition is referred to as a right esophoria. If, with the head turned to the left, the left eye drifts laterally when covered, but shifts medially again to refixate when uncovered, the patient is said to have a left exophoria.

Lower motor neurons in the oculomotor, trochlear, and abducens nuclei function together to ensure that the individual has appropriate and adequate visual access to the world. Most investigators and clinicians recognize three distinct but functionally related types of eye movements: volitional movements, tracking movements, and compensatory or vestibular-driven eye movements. Each of these types of eye movements involves different groups of upper motor neurons, and each can be independently evaluated in the clinical setting. The results of such testing can provide the examiner with valuable information regarding the integrity of different regions of the central nervous system.

Volitional eye movements are used to scan the environment to bring different targets of interest onto the macular portion of the retina. Movements of the head and neck often accompany volitional eye movements as a means of increasing the range or size of the visual world that can be viewed without having to move other parts of the body.

Tracking eye movements are used to maintain fixation on a moving target without the necessity of altering the position of the head or the rest of the body. They are automatic or reflex in nature but can be suppressed by neural activity originating in other areas of the brain. Tracking movements have strong survival value in many animal species, although this need is less prominent in humans.

Compensatory or vestibular-driven eye movements are used to maintain visual fixation on a target when the individual is physically moving in space. Like tracking movements, vestibular-driven eye movements are also reflex in nature but are rarely if ever suppressed. Inappropriate vestibular-driven eye movements may be seen in patients with disease involving the vestibular apparatus or eighth cranial nerve.

Each of these three types of eye movements is controlled to a significant degree by a different area of the central nervous system. Volitional eye movements are controlled from the frontal lobe, tracking eye movements are controlled from the parieto-occipital region, and vestibular-driven eye movements are controlled from nuclei in the pontomedullary region of the brainstem. Each of these regions of the brain influences neurons in an area of the brainstem known as the *paramedian pontine reticular formation* (PPRF), which in turn exerts a controlling influence on the extraocular nuclei. The nature of this controlling influence is to coordinate activity (excitation and inhibition) of the extraocular nuclei so that the resulting eye movements are conjugate and purposeful.

Volitional eye movements are tested by asking the patient to move his or her eyes through the full range in the cardinal planes of motion in response to verbal instructions from the examiner. Normally, the eyes should move promptly and in a conjugate manner. The eyes should be tested both together and separately. Patients with unilateral lesions in the frontal lobe, specifically involving the region of the prefrontal eye fields (Brodmann's area 8) typically have difficulty with tasks requiring voluntary eye movements and perform poorly on tests of volitional eye movements. The ocular motor impairment usually involves both eyes to the same degree. Injuries or disease processes that result in excitation or overactivity of neurons in the prefrontal eye fields are frequently characterized by conjugate deviation of the eyes away from the side of the lesion. In contrast, injuries or disease processes that destroy nerve cells in the prefrontal eye fields reduce the relative influence of that side of the brain on the extraocular nuclei and generally result in paresis or paralysis of gaze to the contralateral side with deviation of the eyes toward the side of the lesion. The conjugate deviation of the eyes toward the side of destructive lesions of the frontal lobe is generally transient, being present in the early stages following injury but resolving shortly thereafter. Patients with unilateral destructive frontal lobe lesions who do not demonstrate tonic deviation of the eyes to the side of the lesion when awake may do so when they are unconscious. Such patients, in addition to having other signs and symptoms associated with frontal lobe lesions, frequently have a gaze paralysis to the uninvolved side.

Tracking eye movements are tested by asking the patient to hold his or her head still and follow the movement of the examiner's finger as it is moved into the six positions indicated in Figure 7. The eyes should follow the movement of the finger smoothly and in a conjugate manner, with no signs of nystagmus, complaints of diplopia, or other indices of ocular motor dysfunction. Injuries or disease processes that impair the normal function of neurons in the parieto-occipital cortex (Brodmann's areas 18 and 19) are characterized by difficulties with visual tracking tasks. Seizures or other lesions involving the parieto-occipital cortex that result in an excitation of the neurons in the region frequently produce a conjugate deviation of the eyes to the opposite side. In addition, patients may experience hallucinations involving flashing lights or peculiar shapes, either stationary or moving in the visual field. Destructive lesions involving the parieto-occipital cortex and the underlying white matter may produce visual tracking deficits, together with a contralateral visual field loss. Difficulties with visual tracking are seen when the eyes must track an object moving from the normal side to the diseased side. For example, a patient with a destructive lesion involving the right parieto-occipital region has difficulty in tracking objects that move from left to right in the visual field, particularly from the position of primary gaze to the right.

Tests of vestibular-driven eye movements are generally performed as part of the evaluation of the vestibulocochlear nerve. A description of specific test procedures and their interpretation will be presented later, together with other tests of vestibulocochlear nerve function.

A particularly important region of the brainstem associated with ocular motor function is the PPRF. Neurons in this region receive synaptic input from a variety of upper motor neuron sources and distribute their axons to all six extraocular nuclei. The PPRF is responsible for the "yoking" together of the abducens nucleus on one side with the oculomotor nucleus of the contralateral side. Nerve fibers involved in these internuclear connections are part of the medial longitudinal fasciculus (MLF). The MLF is the first pathway to myelinate, an indication of its importance.

Lesions can damage the PPRF or the MLF. Unilateral damage to the PPRF produces a paralysis of lateral gaze involving both eyes to the ipsilateral side. When awake, the patient may be able to maintain the eyes in the position of primary gaze, but when asleep or unconscious, a conjugate deviation of the eyes to the contralateral side may be observed. Note that these findings are the reverse of those seen in patients with destructive lesions involving the frontal eye fields.

Lesions involving the MLF are characterized by paralysis of adduction with nystagmus of the abducting eye on lateral gaze. Bilateral internuclear ophthalmoplegia is virtually pathognomonic of multiple sclerosis in individuals between 14 and 45 years of age. Unilateral internuclear ophthalmoplegia is characterized by a paralysis of adduction of the ipsilateral eye with nystagmus in the contralateral abducting eye on lateral gaze to the contralateral side. Unilateral disease in individuals older than 45 years is frequently associated with localized ischemia or infarct involving perforating branches of the basilar artery, which supply the fibers of the MLF in the region of the pons. Clinical findings associated with lesions involving the oculomotor, trochlear, and abducens nerves are easily recognized if the examiner keeps in mind and applies a few simple principles of ocular motor anatomy. Table 7 summarizes the major clinical findings that would be expected in patients with damage to each of these cranial nerves.

TRIGEMINAL NERVE (V)

Functional Anatomy

The trigeminal nerve is a mixed nerve subserving both sensory and motor functions. The nerve conveys general sensory information from the face and scalp, the oral and nasal cavities, part of the meninges, and the cornea. Motor fibers of the trigeminal nerve innervate the muscles of mastication, two muscles of the floor of the mouth, and the tensor tympani muscle.

The cell bodies of the sensory fibers of the trigeminal nerve are located in the trigeminal (gasserian, semilunar) ganglion. This ganglion is

TABLE 7 *Clinical Findings Associated With Ocular Motor Nerve Dysfunction*

Nerve	Major Clinical Findings
Oculomotor (III)	Ptosis that does not resolve with upward gaze Corectasia (mydriasis) Impaired direct and indirect light reflexes in ipsilateral eye Cycloplegia Exotropia with hypotropia Diplopia with attempted lateral gaze to the contralateral side Diplopia for near vision greater than for far vision Intorsion with attempted downward gaze in the abducted position
Trochlear (IV)	Diplopia with attempted downward gaze in the adducted position Head tilt to the contralateral side
Abducens (VI)	Esotropia of the ipsilateral eye Diplopia with attempted lateral gaze to the ipsilateral side Diplopia for far vision greater than for near vision

located immediately adjacent to the posterolateral part of the cavernous sinus in a slight depression in the petrous part of the temporal bone known as Meckel's cave. The peripheral processes of these neurons compose the three divisions of the trigeminal nerve: ophthalmic (V_1), maxillary (V_2), and mandibular (V_3). The ophthalmic division exits the middle cranial fossa by passing through the superior orbital fissure; the maxillary division, by passing through the foramen rotundum; and the mandibular division, by passing through the foramen ovale. The area of skin on the face and scalp innervated by each of the divisions of the trigeminal nerve is illustrated in Figure 8.

The central processes of trigeminal ganglion cells enter the brainstem at the level of the rostral pons and either ascend a short distance to synapse in the principal nucleus of V or descend in the spinal tract of V to terminate in the spinal nucleus of V at pontine, medullary, or upper cervical levels (Fig. 9). Clinical evidence suggests that low-threshold mechanical stimuli, such as are used in the evaluation of light touch and tactile discrimination, are relayed by way of the principal nucleus of V and the most rostral parts of the spinal nucleus of V. In contrast, high-threshold mechanical stimuli, noxious stimuli, and thermal stimuli, all of which are used to evaluate pain and temperature sensibility of the face, are relayed by way of the caudal part (medullary and cervical) of the spinal nucleus of V. Sensation from the cornea is carried in the ophthalmic division of the trigeminal nerve and appears to be relayed by neurons located in the rostral part of the trigeminal nuclear complex.

Nerve cells of the trigeminal nuclear complex are the origin of axons, most of which cross the midline to form the trigeminothalamic pathways. These pathways terminate in a somatotopic fashion in the ventral posteromedial (VPM) nucleus of the thalamus (see Fig. 9). From the thalamus, nerve impulses are relayed by way of the posterior limb of the internal capsule to the postcentral gyrus, where they activate cells in a region near the Sylvian fissure that subserves sensation from the face.

Motor axons carried in the trigeminal nerve innervate the muscles of mastication (masseter, temporalis, medial pterygoid, and lateral pterygoid), two muscles of the floor of the mouth (anterior belly of the digastric and mylohyoid), and the tensor tympani, a muscle that helps to maintain tension on the tympanic membrane. The cell bodies giving rise to motor fibers are located in a small nucleus in the rostral part of the pons known as the motor nucleus of V, or sometimes the masticator nucleus (see Fig. 9). Motor axons leave the cranial cavity by way of the foramen ovale and travel to their target structures in close association with branches of the mandibular nerve.

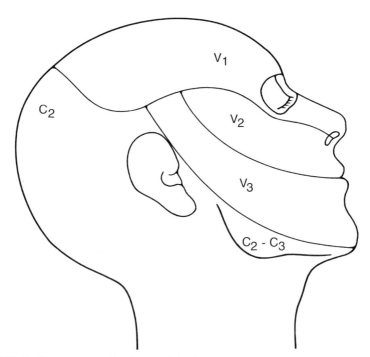

FIGURE 8. The cutaneous distribution of the three divisions of the trigeminal nerve. V_1 = ophthalmic branch, V_2 = maxillary branch, V_3 = mandibular branch. Note that the skin overlying the angle of the mandible is innervated by sensory branches of cervical spinal nerves C_1 and C_3.

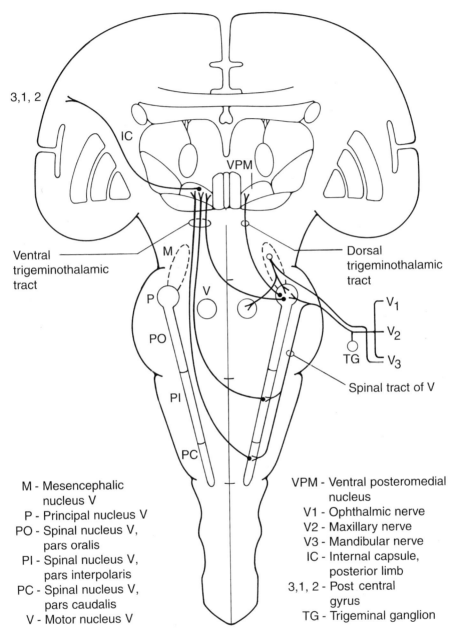

M - Mesencephalic
 nucleus V
P - Principal nucleus V
PO - Spinal nucleus V,
 pars oralis
PI - Spinal nucleus V,
 pars interpolaris
PC - Spinal nucleus V,
 pars caudalis
V - Motor nucleus V

VPM - Ventral posteromedial
 nucleus
V1 - Ophthalmic nerve
V2 - Maxillary nerve
V3 - Mandibular nerve
IC - Internal capsule,
 posterior limb
3,1, 2 - Post central
 gyrus
TG - Trigeminal ganglion

FIGURE 9. Central projections of the trigeminal nerve mediating sensation from the face, including the cornea and mouth. (Modified from Haines, DE: *Neuroanatomy: An Atlas of Structures, Sections, and Systems,* ed 3. Urban & Schwartzenberg, Baltimore and Munich, 1991, with permission.

Afferent neurons involved in position sense of the jaw (proprioception) and the jaw jerk reflex are located not in the trigeminal ganglion, but rather within the brainstem in the mesencephalic nucleus of V (see Fig. 9). Although they are located within the central nervous system, these neurons appear and function like sensory neurons found in the trigeminal ganglion. Their peripheral processes carry information from muscle spindles located in the muscles of mastication. Their central processes synapse on neurons in the principal nucleus of V (proprioception) and the motor nucleus of V (jaw jerk reflex).

Clinical Examinations

Sensory testing of the face can be performed with a safety pin opened so that touch stimuli can be applied with both the sharp and blunt ends. The patient should be made comfortable and asked to close the eyes during testing. Initially, one should touch some area of the patient's skin known to be normal with both the sharp and blunt ends of the pin to acquaint the patient with the two sensations. Sharp and blunt stimuli should be applied in random order to the forehead above the eyebrow, each time giving the patient an opportunity to indicate whether the perceived sensation was sharp or dull. The examiner should note whether the patient has difficulty in distinguishing between the sharp and dull stimuli. When satisfied with the results obtained on one side, the examiner should test the skin of the forehead over the opposite eyebrow in the same manner.

Next, the examiner should apply a sharp stimulus to both sides of the forehead in succession, asking the patient whether the two stimuli feel the same or different. Any discrepancy or difference in the ability to perceive the stimulus on the two sides should be noted. These tests evaluate two phenomena: (1) the ability of the patient to differentiate between sharp and blunt stimuli applied to a particular area of skin and (2) a discrepancy in the perception of sharp stimulation between the two sides of the forehead. After testing the skin of the forehead, which is innervated by fibers carried in the ophthalmic nerve, the examiner should repeat these test procedures on the cheeks over the maxillary prominence (innervated by the maxillary nerve) and on the chin on both sides of the midline near the mental foramen (innervated by the mandibular nerve). When testing sensation mediated by the mandibular division of the trigeminal nerve, avoid touching the skin near the angle of the mandible because this area is innervated by branches of cervical spinal nerves (see Fig. 8).

Reduced sensibility to both sharp and blunt stimulation suggests *hypesthesia* in the distribution of the nerve or nerves tested, whereas reduced or absent sensation to sharp stimulation or the inability to distinguish sharp from blunt stimulation may indicate *hypalgesia*. Increased sensibility to tactile stimulation is described differently, based on the intensity of the stimulus and the patient's perception of its degree of unpleasantness. A greater than normal response to painful stimuli (sharp) is referred to as *hyperalgesia*. A heightened perception to non-noxious stimuli that is not judged to be painful is characterized as *hyperesthesia*, whereas a painful experience resulting from non-noxious stimulation is referred to as *allodynia*.

If altered sensation is suspected, *thermal testing* may be helpful in confirming this suspicion. Thermal testing is performed using test tubes or empty syringe casings filled with warm and cold water. Two test tubes filled with water of the same temperature are placed simultaneously in similar locations on either side of the face, and the patient is asked whether they feel the same or if one feels warmer or cooler than the other. If a discrepancy is noted with warm water in a patient with suspected hypesthesia or hypalgesia, the side that is perceived as warmer is the normal side. If a discrepancy is noted with cold water in a patient with hypesthesia or hypalgesia, the side that is perceived as cooler is the normal side. Thermal testing is not routinely done but should be performed when necessary. It may be uncomfortable in patients with hyperalgesia or allodynia.

The most sensitive test of sensory trigeminal nerve function is the *corneal reflex*. The patient is asked to direct his or her gaze to one side, keeping both eyes open. The examiner then approaches the adducted eye from the lateral side with a wisp of cotton that has been twisted to a point. The examiner touches the cornea over the iris lateral to the pupil, taking care to avoid contacting the conjunctiva or sclera, or passing the cotton tip in front of the pupil. The normal response is an immediate blinking of both eyes, occasionally with movement of the head away from the stimulus. The afferent limb of the corneal reflex is the ophthalmic division of the trigeminal nerve (V_1), and the efferent limb of the reflex is subserved by the facial nerve (VII) (Fig. 10). If damage to the ophthalmic nerve is present, no response will be seen in either eye when the cornea on the involved side is touched. Intact responses in both eyes will be observed when the cornea of the normal eye is touched. In contrast, if a lesion involving the facial nerve is present, no response will be seen on the lesion side when either cornea is touched. The blink response on the nonlesioned side will be present regardless of which cornea is stimulated.

The motor component of the trigeminal nerve innervates the muscles of mastication, the mylohyoid muscle, the anterior belly of the digastric muscle, and the tensor tympani muscle. Of these, only the muscles of mastication are routinely tested in the neurologic examination. The masseter, temporalis, and medial pterygoid muscles function to close the jaw

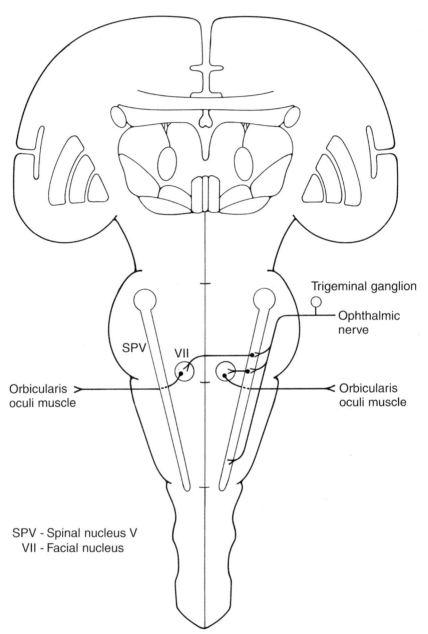

FIGURE 10. The afferent and efferent limbs of the corneal reflex. (Modified from Haines, DE: *Neuroanatomy: An Atlas of Structures, Sections, and Systems*, ed 3. Urban & Schwartzenberg, Baltimore and Munich, 1991, with permission.)

and approximate the molar teeth. The lateral pterygoid muscle functions to protrude and open the jaw.

To test the masseter, temporalis, and medial pterygoid muscles, the patient is asked to close the mouth and gently approximate the molar teeth. With fingers placed on both of the patient's cheeks, the examiner palpates the anterior margin of the masseter. The patient is then asked to alternately bite hard and relax without separating the teeth. As the patient bites down, the examiner palpates the contraction of the masseter on both sides. The muscle contractions should be equal and symmetric. In the normal individual, when the masseter is fully contracting, it will be impossible to separate the jaws by pushing down on the chin. The temporalis muscle can be palpated in the temporal fossa during the same biting maneuver, although its contraction will be less apparent and somewhat more difficult to detect. Patients with loose-fitting or poorly fitting dentures or with tooth pain may have some difficulty with this test or may be reluctant to bite down too hard.

The lateral pterygoid muscle protracts the lower jaw and aids in opening the mouth. It is tested by asking the patient to push the jaw forward with the mouth slightly open. Normally, the jaw moves straight forward approximately 1 cm. Deviation of the jaw to one side suggests weakness or paralysis of the lateral pterygoid on the ipsilateral side.

Although the mylohyoid muscle is not routinely tested, its activity can be easily assessed in the clinical setting. With the patient's jaws relaxed and slightly apart, the examiner gently places his or her fingers bilaterally against the floor of the mouth in the submandibular triangle. The patient is then asked to push the tongue forcefully up against the roof of the mouth. The examiner will be able to palpate the contraction of the mylohyoid. In the normal individual, the contractions should be bilaterally symmetric.

The tensor tympani muscle is not routinely tested in the clinical examination. Patients with trigeminal nerve injuries who lose innervation to this muscle may complain of some difficulty in hearing low-pitched sounds.

FACIAL NERVE (VII)

Functional Anatomy

The facial nerve is a mixed cranial nerve subserving both motor and sensory functions. Motor fibers innervate the muscles of facial expression, including the platysma, the posterior belly of the digastric and stylohyoid muscles, and the stapedius muscle. Sensory fibers transmit taste from the anterior two thirds of the tongue and general sensation from the oropharyngeal mucosa in the region of the palatine tonsils and from a small area of skin in the external ear canal. Autonomic fibers innervate the lacrimal gland, the submandibular and submaxillary salivary glands, and the glands in the nasal mucosa.

The facial nerve emerges from the cerebellomedullary angle and enters the temporal bone by way of the internal acoustic meatus. The intracranial portion of the nerve is composed of two anatomically distinct parts: a comparatively large group of fibers referred to as the facial nerve proper, which provides motor innervation to branchial arch–derived skeletal muscles (facial expression, platysma, stylohyoid, posterior belly of the digastric, and stapedius); and a physically smaller component, the nervus intermedius, which is composed of sensory and autonomic fibers (Fig. 11).

The cell bodies of the motor axons lie in the caudal pons in the facial nucleus. The nucleus is located in the ventrolateral part of the pontine tegmentum, a fact which helps explain the peculiar intra-axial location and course of its axons. Within the temporal bone, the motor axons course posteriorly medial to the middle ear structures and then inferiorly to exit the skull via the stylomastoid foramen. Within the vertical portion of the facial canal, the nerve gives off a small branch that innervates the stapedius muscle.

On exiting the stylomastoid foramen, the nerve divides into three small branches: the posterior auricular nerve, which provides motor innervation to the occipitalis muscle and superior and posterior auricular muscles; and two smaller nerve branches, which innervate the posterior belly of the digastric and stylohyoid muscles. The remaining fibers enter the parotid gland, divide into the temporofacial and cervicofacial divisions of the nerve, and further divide into five terminal branches (temporal, zygomatic, buccal, mandibular, and cervical), which innervate the muscles of facial expression (see Fig. 11).

The cell bodies of the sensory component of the facial nerve form the geniculate ganglion, which lies in the petrous part of the temporal bone, several millimeters lateral to the internal acoustic meatus. The peripheral processes innervate taste buds located ipsilaterally on the anterior two thirds of the tongue. Axons conveying taste course with the lingual nerve in the mouth and the chorda tympani in the middle ear and ultimately join the motor axons of the facial nerve at a point just above the stylomastoid foramen in the vertical portion of the facial canal. The central processes of these special sensory neurons reach the brainstem as part of the nervus intermedius. The axons enter the tractus solitarius, where some of them descend for a short distance before finally terminating in the rostral part of the nucleus solitarius (Fig. 12). Because the rostral part of the nucleus solitarius receives synaptic contacts from neurons innervating taste buds, it is sometimes referred to as the gustatory nucleus. (Later we will see that the glossopharyngeal nerve and the vagus nerve also contain taste fibers, and these also terminate in the rostral part of the nucleus solitarius).

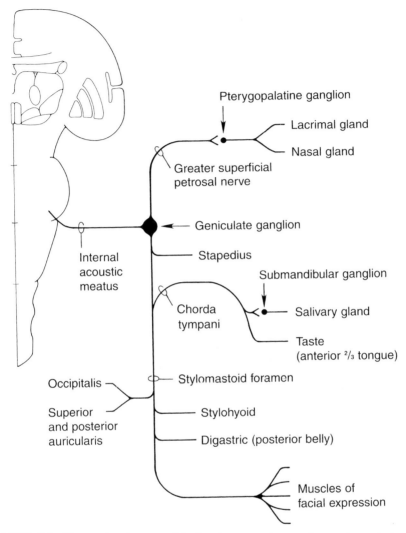

FIGURE 11. The peripheral course of the facial nerve, indicating the muscles and glands innervated. (Modified from Haines, DE: *Neuroanatomy: An Atlas of Structures, Sections, and Systems,* ed 3. Urban & Schwartzenberg, Baltimore and Munich, 1991, with permission.)

A small number of neurons in the geniculate ganglion subserve sensation from skin in the external auditory canal. The peripheral processes course with the facial nerve and are distributed to the region of the external ear canal by way of branches of the posterior auricular nerve. The central processes of these somatic afferent fibers, like those conveying taste, reach the brainstem as part of the nervus intermedius. Unlike the fibers subserving taste, however, which terminate in the nucleus solita-

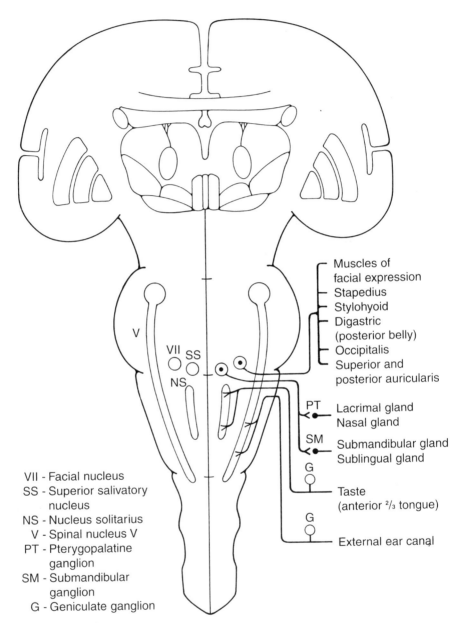

FIGURE 12. The central nuclei and peripheral ganglia associated with the facial nerve. (Modified from Haines, DE: *Neuroanatomy: An Atlas of Structures, Sections, and Systems,* ed 3. Urban & Schwartzenberg, Baltimore and Munich, 1991, with permission.)

rius, the central processes of somatic afferent fibers enter the spinal tract of V, where they descend a short distance before terminating in the spinal nucleus of V (see Fig. 12). (*Note:* An organizational feature of sensory nuclei in the brainstem, which is suggested here and will be highlighted again when we consider cranial nerves IX and X, is that the central processes of visceral afferent neurons terminate in the nucleus solitarius or its rostral part, the gustatory nucleus, whereas the central processes of somatic afferent neurons terminate in the spinal nucleus of V).

The autonomic (parasympathetic) component of the facial nerve provides motor innervation to the lacrimal gland, the submandibular and submaxillary salivary glands, and glands in the nasal mucosa. The preganglionic parasympathetic nerve cell bodies are located at the level of the pontomedullary junction in the superior salivatory nucleus (see Fig. 12). The axons leave the brainstem and pass through the internal acoustic meatus as part of the nervus intermedius. At the lateral end of the internal acoustic meatus, in the region of the geniculate ganglion, the preganglionic parasympathetic fibers divide into two bundles, one coursing anteriorly as part of the greater superficial petrosal nerve, and the other coursing posteriorly with the motor fibers of the facial nerve (see Fig. 11).

The axons that join the greater superficial petrosal nerve course through the pterygoid (Vidian) canal to reach the pterygopalatine fossa, where they make synaptic contact with postganglionic parasympathetic neurons in the pterygopalatine ganglion. Axons arising from these parasympathetic ganglion cells course with the nasociliary and lacrimal branches of the ophthalmic nerve to reach the orbit and lacrimal gland and with branches of the maxillary division of the trigeminal nerve to reach glands in the mucosa of the nasal cavity.

The axons that course posteriorly from the geniculate ganglion in the company of motor fibers of the facial nerve separate from the nerve a short distance above the stylomastoid foramen and join with taste fibers in the chorda tympani. These preganglionic parasympathetic axons leave the chorda tympani in the infratemporal fossa and course with the lingual branch of the mandibular nerve to make synaptic contact with neurons in the submandibular ganglion, located in the floor of the mouth. Short postganglionic parasympathetic axons originating from neurons in the submandibular ganglion distribute to the submandibular and sublingual glands to induce salivation.

Because of the anatomic organization of the facial nerve, lesions at different points along its course would be expected to produce different signs and symptoms, depending on the nerve fibers involved. Careful attention to the symptoms reported by the patient, together with skill in evaluating each functional component of the nerve, in most cases permits the clinician to determine the site of nerve injury precisely.

Clinical Examinations

Assessment of facial nerve function should begin with the examiner carefully observing the patient's face, paying particular attention to the lower eyelids, nasolabial folds, and corners of the mouth. In neurologically intact individuals, the face should appear essentially symmetric. Obvious asymmetries may result from habit, faulty dental occlusion, or trauma, however, and do not necessarily indicate neurologic disease. Patients with unilateral damage to the facial nerve may demonstrate slight drooping of the lower eyelid, possibly with tears appearing on the cheek (epiphora), flattening of the nasolabial fold, and drooping of the corner of the mouth on the affected side. Saliva may dribble from the corner of the mouth, and the patient may be observed repeatedly wiping the face with a handkerchief to prevent the embarrassment of this dribbling. Speech may be slurred to a greater or lesser degree because of weakness or paralysis of the perioral muscles. Also, the eye on the involved side might not fully close with blinking or voluntary eye closure.

Not all of the muscles of facial expression need to be tested individually. The following test maneuvers are sufficient to evaluate the integrity of the nerve. First, ask the patient to hold the head steady, look upward, and raise the eyebrows. Contraction of the frontalis muscle should produce wrinkles in the forehead. In patients with lesions involving the facial nerve, the eyebrow on the involved side may not rise and no wrinkles will appear on that side. Next, ask the patient to close both eyes forcefully. The examiner should gently try to pry the eyes open. In normal individuals, eye closure should be symmetric and of equal strength even if facial features appear to be asymmetric. In a patient with facial nerve dysfunction, the approximation of the upper and lower eyelids will be incomplete or will fail (lagophthalmos). Forceful eye closure is accompanied by supraduction of the eye (Bell's phenomenon). In patients who are unable to approximate the eyelids, the sclera below the iris will be seen between the eyelids.

The patient should then be asked to smile widely, showing the teeth. When the facial nerve is damaged, the corner of the mouth on the involved side will not move laterally and the smile will be asymmetric. Next, ask the patient to purse the lips as if attempting to whistle or kiss. Patients with lesions involving the facial nerve will be unable to bring the lips together on the involved side. Muscle weakness involving the muscles of the lower part of the face may become more apparent if the patient is asked to alternate quickly between smiling and pursing the lips.

The platysma muscle may be difficult to test; a variety of methods have been proposed to help the patient contract this muscle. One that may be useful is to ask the patient to protrude the chin and smile widely. However, the inability to contract the platysma muscle in the absence of other indicators of facial nerve dysfunction should not necessarily be taken as evidence of damage to the cervical branches of the facial nerve. Some individuals may have poorly developed platysma muscles, and others may simply be unable to contract the muscle voluntarily. Caution is therefore necessary when interpreting tests of platysma muscle function.

Occasionally patients present with an inability to close one eye fully but have no other clinical evidence of facial nerve injury. Recall that the afferent limb of the corneal reflex is the ophthalmic division of the trigeminal nerve and that the efferent limb is the facial nerve. Keep in mind also that both eyes close when one eye is threatened. If the facial nerve is involved, the eye on the involved side will not blink when either cornea is stimulated. Closure of the eye in response to corneal stimulation on either or both sides is persuasive evidence against the presence of facial nerve damage. If, however, neither eye closes in response to stimulation of the left cornea, and the left eye does not close voluntarily or to stimulation of the right cornea, it is possible that the patient has a lesion or lesions involving (in this case) both the left trigeminal nerve and the left facial nerve. The left eye would be both unprotected as a result of facial nerve damage and anesthetic as a result of trigeminal nerve damage, a situation that places the eye and vision at considerable risk.

The facial nerve conveys chemical (taste) stimuli from the anterior two thirds of the tongue. Taste is tested by applying dilute solutions of glucose (sweet), sodium chloride (salty), citric acid (sour), and quinine (bitter) to either side of the tongue separately by means of a cotton applicator dipped in the test solution. The patient should be given a card or a piece of paper on which the words SWEET, SALTY, SOUR, BITTER, and WATER are clearly written. The tongue should be extended from the mouth. If necessary, it can be held out by the examiner, who may grasp the tongue with a small gauze pad. A cotton applicator moistened with the test solution should be gently rubbed on one side of the tongue while the patient points to the word indicating the taste perceived. Both sides of the tongue should be tested separately. Quinine should be used last because it may leave an aftertaste. The patient should be permitted to rinse the tongue and mouth thoroughly with water after each stimulus application. Water should be used as a control stimulus to see whether the patient is malingering or faking a disease condition. Patients with damage to the taste fibers carried in the facial nerve may point to the word "water" when one of the other test substances is applied to the tongue.

The absence of taste (ageusia) unilaterally or bilaterally or reduced taste sensation (hypogeusia) can be seen with lesions involving the facial nerve anywhere along its intracranial or intraosseous course. Lesions involving the chorda tympani branch of the facial nerve or the lingual nerve distal to the point where the fibers of the chorda tympani join it may also cause an ipsilateral loss or decrement in taste sensation.

The autonomic (parasympathetic) component of the facial nerve, which provides motor innervation to the lacrimal gland and the salivary glands, is not routinely tested. If necessary, lacrimal gland function can be tested by placing a narrow strip of litmus paper in the conjunctival space between the sclera and the lower eyelid. Testing should be performed simultaneously in both eyes, noting the rate at which the litmus paper becomes moist. Damage to the facial nerve or the greater superficial petrosal nerve may cause a loss of lacrimation in the ipsilateral eye. Patients with lesions that denervate the lacrimal gland may complain about pain or discomfort in the eye with blinking.

Clinical findings commonly associated with lesions involving the facial nerve include an inability to completely close the eye, drooping of the corner of the mouth, and difficulty with speech articulation. Some patients may complain of dryness of the eye, causing discomfort associated with blinking or eye movements beneath a partially closed eyelid. A particularly bothersome problem is that saliva may drip from the mouth and food may remain in the buccal cavity (cheek pouch) when the patient is eating. Collectively, these problems can profoundly affect the psychological and social well-being of the patient.

Some patients may complain that their hearing seems to be different in one ear or that ambient sounds cause some degree of discomfort or pain. Lesions involving the facial nerve can impair the function of the stapedius muscle, eliminating the dampening effect this muscle exerts on the movement of the stapes in the oval window. The result will be increased movement of the ear ossicles in response to auditory stimuli and a louder-than-normal perception of sound in that ear (hyperacusis).

The most common site of injury involving the facial nerve is at or near the stylomastoid foramen as the nerve exits the skull. Damage to the nerve in this location causes a facial paralysis involving all of the muscles on the ipsilateral side of the face, a condition referred to as *Bell's palsy*. If the lesion is slightly more proximal along the course of the nerve, at a location proximal to the origin of the chorda tympani, the patient may present with ageusia in addition to weakness or paralysis of the facial muscles. If the lesion is in the internal ear canal or in the region of the internal acoustic meatus, the patient may demonstrate reduced function of the lacrimal gland on that side along with ageusia and Bell's palsy. Usually, both the presence and site of a lesion involving the facial nerve can be determined with confidence based on the history and clinical findings. The clinical evaluation of the facial nerve is, in essence, an exercise in applied anatomy.

Lesions involving the corticobulbar projections to the facial nucleus produce different, though equally characteristic, clinical findings. Unilateral lesions involving corticobulbar axons as they course through the internal capsule, midbrain, or pons produce a contralateral facial weakness involving only the muscles of the lower half of the face (Fig. 13). Smiling and lip pursing will be impaired contralateral to the side of the lesion, while the

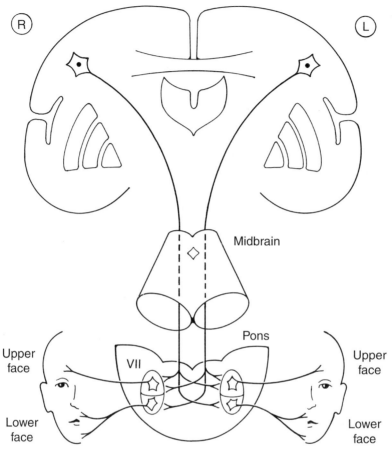

FIGURE 13. Corticonuclear projections to the facial nucleus. (Modified from Haines, DE: *Neuroanatomy: An Atlas of Structures, Sections, and Systems,* ed 3. Urban & Schwartzenberg, Baltimore and Munich, 1991, with permission.)

ability to close the eyes and wrinkle the forehead will be essentially intact. Interestingly, some patients who are unable to smile symmetrically on request can do so in response to a funny story or humorous comment. This observation suggests that cortical influences on lower motor neurons of the facial nucleus may originate from more than one area of the cerebral cortex.

VESTIBULOCOCHLEAR NERVE (VIII)

The vestibulocochlear nerve is composed of two functionally distinct components or divisions. The cochlear division is concerned with audition, the sense and experience of hearing. The vestibular division is concerned with equilibrium. More specifically, the vestibular system is involved in monitoring the position and orientation of the head in space while we are stationary and as we move about.

Cochlear Nerve

Functional Anatomy

The cell bodies of the cochlear nerve compose the spiral ganglion and are located in the bony modiolus of the cochlea (Fig. 14). The short, peripheral processes of these cells innervate specialized receptor cells found in the organ of Corti, located within the petrous part of the temporal bone. The central processes, which constitute the cochlear nerve, enter the middle cranial fossa by way of the internal acoustic meatus and reach the cerebellomedullary angle, where they make synaptic contact with neurons in the dorsal and ventral cochlear nuclei. The anatomic organization of central auditory pathways originating from the cochlear nuclei is complex and is not addressed in great detail here. For our purposes, it is sufficient to remember that auditory impulses are carried rostrally to the inferior colliculus in the lateral lemniscus, and that auditory information from one ear is carried largely in the contralateral lateral lemniscus. From the inferior colliculus, auditory impulses are relayed to the medial geniculate nucleus and then, by way of the sublenticular part of the internal capsule, to the superior transverse temporal gyrus (Heschl's convolution, Brodmann's area 41). While perception of sound occurs in Heschl's convolution, the interpretation of auditory stimuli involves nerve cells in the nearby auditory association areas (Brodmann's areas 42 and 22) of the temporal lobe.

Clinical Examinations

Tests of auditory function range from the simple to the complex; the test used depends on the clinical situation. The more simple tests are generally adequate for patients who do not complain of hearing impairment and should be performed as part of the routine neurologic examination. At other times, a more thorough assessment of auditory function may be necessary, although the more complex tests often require specialized equipment that may not be readily available. When used, however, these tests can provide detailed and valuable information on hearing ability. They may be particularly useful in quantifying hearing change over time or as it may be affected by disease progression or therapeutic intervention. Patients who indicate difficulty in hearing conversations over the telephone or who favor one ear over the other when talking on the tele-

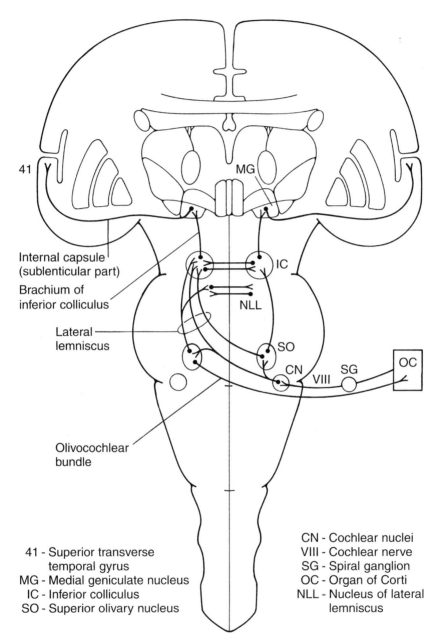

FIGURE 14. The peripheral and central auditory pathways. (Modified from Haines, DE: *Neuroanatomy: An Atlas of Structures, Sections, and Systems,* ed 3. Urban & Schwartzenberg, Baltimore and Munich, 1991, with permission.)

phone are telling you that they may be experiencing some sort of hearing deficit.

The first requirement for auditory testing is a quiet environment, free from noise and other auditory distractions. Achieving a quiet environment for testing is sometimes the most difficult part of the examination and is sometimes overlooked even by the most experienced clinician, but it should be the number one priority in preparing to test auditory function.

The next most important part of the auditory examination is to inspect the external ear canal and the tympanic membrane. An otoscope with an appropriate speculum should be used for this purpose. The ear canal must be free of obstruction. Cerumen or other foreign material in the ear canal should be carefully removed by appropriate means, taking care to avoid impacting foreign substances against the tympanic membrane or damaging the membrane itself. The tympanic membrane should also be thoroughly inspected for tears and displacement, both of which can alter or impair hearing ability. Middle ear infections may cause fluid or pus to accumulate behind the tympanic membrane; these may be visible through the eardrum or cause it to bulge outward. The presence of such material in the middle ear cavity can limit the movement of the ossicles and thereby impair hearing. Any abnormalities detected by visual inspection should be adequately documented in the patient's record.

A simple test of auditory function is for the examiner to rub his or her fingers together at some distance lateral to the patient's ear. The starting point should be far enough away that an individual with normal hearing will not be able to detect the sound. The examiner should be positioned directly in front of the patient so that the examiner's own hearing can be used as a control. The examiner slowly moves the fingers toward the patient's ear, asking the patient to indicate when the sound is first heard. Hearing ability for that ear is documented by recording the distance between the examiner's fingers and the patient's ear when the rubbing sound is first heard. After one ear is tested, the procedure should be repeated on the other side. Some practice will be required to ensure consistency in the intensity of the rubbing noise used and to establish the distance measures that represent normal hearing. As a general rule, most persons with normal hearing should be able to hear the rubbing noise at a distance of approximately 20 to 24 inches.

Further testing is necessary in patients who perform poorly on this simple screening test or who complain of hearing impairment. The *Rinne test* is useful for distinguishing conduction deficits from sensorineural deficits in patients who complain of reduced hearing (hypacusis) or absent hearing (anacusis). The test is performed by placing the base of a vibrating tuning fork (256 or 512 Hz) against the mastoid process. The patient is asked to indicate when the tone is no longer heard. At that moment, the tines of the tuning fork are brought close to the external auditory meatus, and the patient is asked if the tone is heard again. In an individual with normal hearing, the tone will be heard again and will continue to be heard for about twice as long as was the case for the sound transmitted by bone conduction. The normal response is documented as "AC > BC."

A patient with sensorineural hearing loss will also hear the tone again, but the duration of the tone perceived by air conduction will be reduced. In this case, the Rinne test is said to be "positive," and the results are reported as "AC > BC" for that ear. It is useful in cases like this to document as accurately as possible the length of time the tone was heard by both bone and air conduction, and to include a note in the patient's chart indicating that the decreased hearing times are suggestive of cochlear nerve damage.

In patients with obstruction of the external ear canal or disease of the middle ear that restricts the movement of the auditory ossicles, the tone will not return when the tines are brought close to the ear. The Rinne test in this case would be considered "negative," and the results would be documented as "BC > AC" for that ear. Conditions in which BC > AC are characterized as conduction deafness. The Rinne test should be performed on both sides in all patients with suspected monaural or binaural hearing loss.

Additional evidence regarding the nature of a hearing deficit can be obtained by means of the *Weber test.* The test is performed by placing the base of the tuning fork on the vertex of the skull or in the center of the forehead. The patient is asked to indicate on which side, if either, the tone is louder. An individual with normal hearing will report that the tone is heard equally on both sides. A patient with unilateral sensorineural hearing loss will indicate that the tone is louder in the normal ear; that is, the tone is lateralized to the good ear. The Weber test results would be reported as "negative," indicating that the tone is lateralized to the uninvolved side. A patient with unilateral conduction deafness will report that the tone is louder on the diseased side; that is, the tone is lateralized to the bad ear. The test result would be reported as "positive," indicating that the tone is lateralized to the involved side.

Many clinicians suggest that a tuning fork vibrating at 256 Hz should be used to perform the Rinne and Weber tests, but others recommend 512 Hz.

Hearing impairments may be found in association with a number of neurologic conditions and disease processes. Hearing loss that occurs with aging (presbycusis) may come on gradually, typically involves both ears equally, and may go unnoticed until it is brought to the attention of the individual. Such hearing losses involve high-frequency tones first and can be easily detected by simple methods such as finger rubbing. It is therefore important to examine hearing in all patients, particularly those aged 50 years and older.

Approximately 50% of patients who have suffered a stroke in the distribution of the middle cerebral artery have an increased auditory threshold on the hemiplegic side. Many of these patients may have a subtle hearing loss on that side. Tinnitus—a hissing, roaring, whistling, or humming in the ear—may be found in patients with otosclerosis and may or may not be accompanied by a hearing loss. Patients with Ménière's disease may have a hearing loss together with tinnitus, vertigo, and nystagmus. Hypacusis also is often seen in patients with acoustic neuromas. It is therefore important to evaluate auditory function carefully in any patient with a hearing problem.

Vestibular Nerve

Functional Anatomy

The vestibular division of the eighth cranial nerve transmits nerve impulses from specialized receptor cells located in the semicircular canals, utricle, and saccule. The receptors in the semicircular canals respond to rotational movements of the head (angular displacement), and those in the utricle and saccule are most responsive to movements of the head in a particular direction (linear displacement). As a consequence of the anatomic organization and placement of these receptor cells, it should be apparent that movement in any plane or about any axis will more or less selectively excite certain receptors on one side of the head and inhibit other receptors on the contralateral side of the head. This fact is useful to keep in mind when thinking about the rationale behind specific test procedures for vestibular function.

The nerve cell bodies of the vestibular nerve are located close to the receptor cells in the vestibular (Scarpa's) ganglion (Fig. 15). The central processes enter the middle cranial fossa by way of the internal auditory meatus and reach the brainstem at the cerebellomedullary angle, in close association with the axons of the cochlear division of the nerve. On entering the brainstem, most fibers synapse in the vestibular nuclei. A small number of fibers course in the juxtarestiform body to enter the cerebellum, where they make synaptic contact with nerve cells in the cortex of the flocculonodular lobe.

The axons of nerve cells in the vestibular nuclei distribute widely to nuclear areas in the spinal cord, brainstem, and forebrain. Table 8 is a simplified overview of some of the functions mediated by particular vestibular projection pathways, and some of the signs and symptoms that might be seen when the vestibular nerve or receptors are damaged.

Vestibular function is usually evaluated only when there are signs of

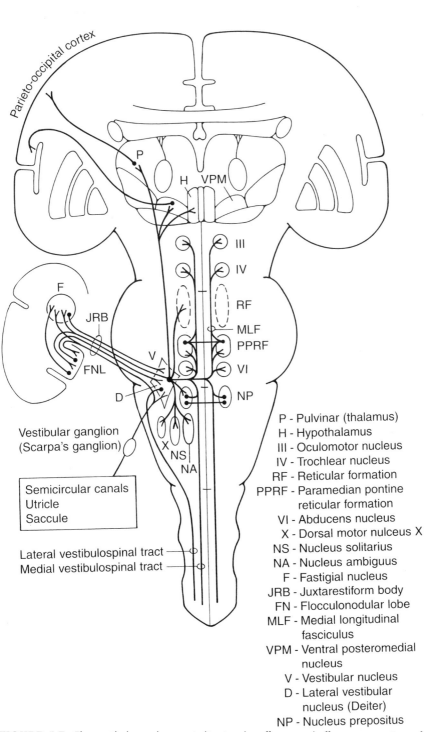

P - Pulvinar (thalamus)
H - Hypothalamus
III - Oculomotor nucleus
IV - Trochlear nucleus
RF - Reticular formation
PPRF - Paramedian pontine
reticular formation
VI - Abducens nucleus
X - Dorsal motor nulceus X
NS - Nucleus solitarius
NA - Nucleus ambiguus
F - Fastigial nucleus
JRB - Juxtarestiform body
FN - Flocculonodular lobe
MLF - Medial longitudinal
fasciculus
VPM - Ventral posteromedial
nucleus
V - Vestibular nucleus
D - Lateral vestibular
nucleus (Deiter)
NP - Nucleus prepositus

FIGURE 15. The vestibular pathways, indicating the afferent and efferent connections of the vestibular nuclei. (Modified from Haines, DE: *Neuroanatomy: An Atlas of Structures, Sections, and Systems*, ed 3. Urban & Schwartzenberg, Baltimore and Munich, 1991, with permission.)

TABLE 8   *Summary of Clinically Important Functions of the Vestibular Nerve*

Projection	Function	Sign	Symptom
Extraocular nuclei	Control of eye movements	Nystagmus	Oscillopsia
Parieto-occipital cortex	Conscious experience of orientation in space		Vertigo
Dorsal motor nucleus of X	GI control	Vomiting	
Nucleus solitarius			Nausea
Spinal cord	Support against gravity	Falling	
Reticular formation	Autonomic control	Facial pallor, sweating	

GI = gastrointestinal.

vestibular disease or complaints that might be attributable to vestibular or cerebellar dysfunction. When signs or symptoms of vestibular dysfunction are suggested in the history, the examiner should begin by asking about and looking carefully for other signs and symptoms of vestibular disease that might have been overlooked. Careful observation and inquiry may be needed because signs and symptoms associated with certain disease processes affecting vestibular function may wax and wane over time or may appear only during certain activities or only when the head or eyes are in certain positions. In any case, a full characterization of signs and symptoms related to vestibular function is necessary before specific tests are performed to rule out or establish the presence of vestibular disease. The list of signs and symptoms in Table 8 should be useful in determining the likelihood of some sort of vestibular disease.

Clinical Examinations

We will first describe simple tests and their interpretation and then move on to more complicated procedures. The order of presentation represents one way of proceeding in an organized manner and is not intended to suggest which test procedures are more or less likely to be of value in diagnosing vestibular disease.

The past-pointing test is performed by asking the patient to alternately touch his or her nose and reach toward the examiner's finger. The examiner places his or her finger directly in front of the patient, just beyond the patient's arm length. Patients should be asked to repeat this maneuver three or four times with their eyes open and then continue to do so after closing their eyes. It is preferable that the patient not actually touch the examiner's finger, so that when the movement is done with the eyes closed, the patient does not keep the arm outstretched searching for the examiner's finger or get the impression that the object of the test is to touch the examiner's finger. An individual with normal vestibular function will be able to alternately touch his or her nose and reach forward and come within a reasonable distance of the examiner's finger with the eyes closed. Patients with unilateral vestibular disease characterized by a re-duced vestibular input from one side will demonstrate a drift away from the examiner's finger toward the side of the vestibular disease when reaching forward with the eyes closed. Both the right and left hand should be tested, and the observed drift with either hand should be con-sistently toward the diseased side. The chart record for a patient who demonstrates drifting to the right, for example, should read "past-point-ing tests show drifting to the right with both hands."

Another test that might be used to evaluate vestibular function is to have the patient march in place with the eyes open and then closed. Nor-mal individuals continue to face in the same direction whether their eyes are open or closed. Patients with vestibular disease tend to rotate to one side when the eyes are closed. Patients with vestibular disease may also report dizziness or vertigo when they march with their eyes closed. Oth-ers may stumble to one side or fall to the diseased side. Any rotation will be toward the side of the nonfunctioning vestibular apparatus, and its di-rection should be documented in the patient's chart. The chart note for a patient who turns to the right while marching in place should read "rota-tion to the right while marching in place."

Oscillopsia (the experience that objects in the visual field seem to be wiggling or moving back and forth) and nystagmus (rapid linear or rota-tory movements of the eye) are common findings in diseases affecting the vestibular apparatus. Both must be thoroughly evaluated when present or carefully looked for if not detected or continuously evident. Many kinds of nystagmus have been described in the literature. For our pur-poses, we can reduce them to three fundamental types: those induced by eye position (gaze nystagmus), head position (positional nystagmus), or head movement.

Gaze nystagmus is produced when the eyes are in the position of pri-mary gaze or are shifted in a particular direction. Tests for gaze nystag-mus simply involve having the patient look straight ahead or shift the gaze in one direction and then another. Gaze need not be shifted by more than 30 degrees in any direction because moving further from the posi-tion of primary gaze may induce nystagmus even in normal individuals. Gaze nystagmus is typically biphasic, with a fast phase (for which the nystagmus is named) and a slow phase. For example, a horizontal nystag-mus in which the eyes move slowly to the left and then rapidly back to the right would be referred to as a right nystagmus. The slow component is driven by vestibular mechanisms, and the rapid, resetting response in the opposite direction is cortically mediated. Patients who present with gaze nystagmus always demonstrate the fast component in the direction of gaze. Such patients may also complain of oscillopsia when they shift their gaze in the direction that produces nystagmus. These findings may suggest damage to the vestibular nuclei or system on the contralateral side. Patients should be tested for gaze nystagmus in all directions, and positive findings should be clearly documented in the patient chart. For example, the note on a patient who demonstrates a left nystagmus on looking to the left should read "left nystagmus with left lateral gaze." This observation would suggest vestibular disease on the right side.

Sometimes the degree of nystagmus can be subtle. The use of Frenzel glasses (lenses of +20 diopters) may be helpful in these cases because they prevent patients from being able to focus their vision and they also magnify the eye and pupil so that small movements can be more easily seen by the examiner.

Positional nystagmus occurs when the head assumes a particular position or orientation in space. Patients with positional nystagmus are generally more troubled by the experience of vertigo, which commonly occurs with particular head positions. The *Nylen-Bárány maneuver* or one of its variants are commonly used to evaluate complaints of vertigo and positional nystagmus. The test is performed by rapidly shifting the patient from the sitting to the backlying position, while at the same time turning the patient's head to the right or left. The head movement should come to a stop at a position below the level of the table or bed. The patient may be asked to direct his or her gaze in the direction of the head rotation, but this is not necessary. Having lowered the patient and turned the patient's head, the examiner looks for nystagmus, which may take several seconds to develop, and inquires as to whether the patient experiences vertigo. The test is designed to assess the function of the utricle on the side closest to the floor. It is considered "positive" if the patient develops nystagmus to the side of that ear. Patients with acute labyrinthitis generally become quite dizzy during this maneuver and frequently close their eyes in an attempt to overcome this feeling. Gross body movements may also occur, and the examiner must firmly support the patient, who may be fearful as a result of disequilibrium. A positive response to the Nylen-Bárány test is dramatic, and the examiner will have little difficulty in recognizing it when it occurs. The test should be performed twice, once turning the head in each direction. Several minutes should be allowed between tests to permit fluid movement in the receptor apparatus to stop, and to allow any vertigo to disappear. The chart record should describe the responses seen with turning the head both to the right and to the left, including the direction and duration of the induced nystagmus and whether or not the patient experienced vertigo or nausea.

The functional integrity of the vestibular receptors and system can also be assessed by means of *caloric testing*. For this test, the patient should be placed comfortably in the supine position with the neck flexed approximately 30 degrees from the horizontal position. The head should be supported with a pillow. The ear to be tested should be carefully examined with an otoscope to ensure that the tympanic membrane is intact. Frank middle-ear disease or tears in the eardrum are contraindications for caloric testing. Ten milliters of ice water are gently instilled into the external ear canal over the course of about 10 seconds. A device consisting of a flexible piece of tubing attached to a syringe can be used for this purpose. The tubing should fit comfortably in the external ear canal with the opening placed several millimeters from the tympanic membrane. The tubing should be small enough in external diameter to permit the water to escape the ear canal during irrigation, and care must be exercised to avoid damaging the eardrum by the force of water pressure. The procedure should not be unduly uncomfortable for the patient.

The normal response to infusion of ice water should be a biphasic, horizontal nystagmus with the fast component to the opposite side. The response may take several seconds to appear and may last several seconds following irrigation. A horizontal nystagmus is produced because of convection currents set up in the horizontal canal, which is in the vertical position by virtue of the position of the head. Cold-induced lymphokinesis inhibits the receptor cells in the irrigated horizontal canal, which in turn causes a contralateral nystagmus and past-pointing to the ipsilateral or irrigated side. If a normal individual is tested by means of the past-pointing test immediately after irrigation with ice water, the arms will be seen to drift to the irrigated side.

Patients with a nonfunctioning vestibular apparatus or complete vestibular nerve damage will not respond to caloric stimulation on that side, a condition referred to as *canal paresis*. Asymmetric responses in the two eyes suggest a pontine lesion, disease involving the medial longitudinal fasciculus, or lesions involving the extraocular nuclei or nerves.

A response in which the eyes are tonically deviated toward the side of the cold-irrigated ear suggests bilateral cerebral disease. The explanation for this observation is that unilateral irrigation with cold water in the normal individual causes a reduction in vestibular input to the central nervous system from that side. The relative increase in excitation from the nonirrigated contralateral side results in a vestibular-driven deviation of the eyes to the cold-irrigated side. Cortical influences in the neurologically intact individual cause a rapid deviation of the eyes in the opposite direction — that is, away from the cold-irrigated side. Unilateral irrigation with cold water in the normal individual, therefore, results in contralateral nystagmus. If the cortical component is absent (as in coma), the fast, cortically driven movement to the contralateral side is lost, but the slow, vestibular-driven deviation to the irrigated side will be retained. For this reason, caloric testing can be useful in evaluating brainstem function in the unconscious patient.

Caloric testing, when indicated, should be performed on both sides. A patient with a normal response to caloric stimulation on one side and no response following irrigation of the other side is likely to have unilateral vestibular disease on the side that did not evoke a response. The chart record should fully describe the response seen with irrigation of each ear: whether or not a response to caloric stimulation was seen; the direction of the induced nystagmus, if present; some indication of the time of onset and completion of the response relative to the irrigation; and any vertigo or nausea the patient experiences.

It is very important for the inexperienced examiner to realize that some of these procedures, particularly the Nylen-Bárány and caloric tests, can provoke anxiety or discomfort in patients, especially if they are already discomforted by their disease. The examiner should make every effort to explain the purpose of these tests before performing them, to put patients at rest and gain their confidence in his or her clinical ability. It is often surprising how a little attention to the spoken or unspoken concerns and apprehensions of the patient can make the clinical evaluation less unpleasant for the patient and more productive for the examiner.

GLOSSOPHARYNGEAL NERVE (IX)

Functional Anatomy

The glossopharyngeal nerve is a mixed nerve subserving both motor and sensory functions. The efferent (motor) fibers are of two types: one originating from nerve cells in the nucleus ambiguus and the other originating in the inferior salivatory nucleus (Fig. 16). Axons originating in the nucleus ambiguus emerge from the brainstem immediately dorsal to the inferior olive at its rostral end. From there, they course toward the jugular foramen and pass through it to exit the skull. These fibers provide motor innervation to the stylopharyngeus muscle, the only skeletal muscle innervated by the glossopharyngeal nerve. The inferior salivatory nucleus contains preganglionic parasympathetic nerve cell bodies. The axons of these cells leave the skull by way of the jugular foramen and make synaptic contact with postganglionic parasympathetic neurons located in the otic ganglion. Postganglionic parasympathetic fibers originating in the otic ganglion innervate the parotid gland.

Afferent fibers of the glossopharyngeal nerve are also of two types: visceral and somatic. Visceral afferent fibers convey sensation from the pharyngeal mucosa, taste from the posterior third of the tongue, and impulses from the baroreceptors in the carotid sinus. The nerve cell bodies of these visceral afferent fibers are located immediately outside the jugu-

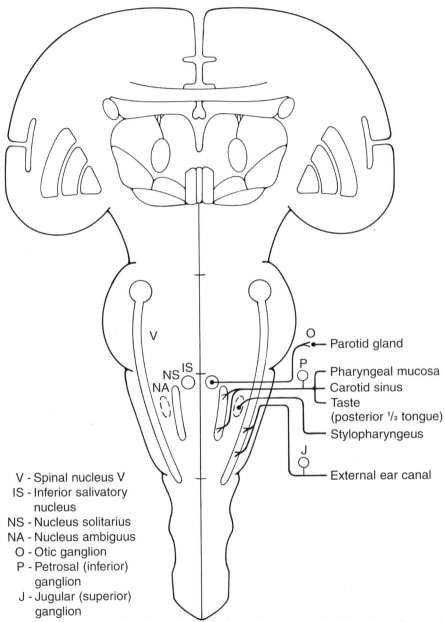

V - Spinal nucleus V
IS - Inferior salivatory
      nucleus
NS - Nucleus solitarius
NA - Nucleus ambiguus
O - Otic ganglion
P - Petrosal (inferior)
      ganglion
J - Jugular (superior)
      ganglion

FIGURE 16. The central nuclei and peripheral ganglia associated with the glossopharyngeal nerve (IX). (Modified from Haines, DE: *Neuroanatomy: An Atlas of Structures, Sections, and Systems*, ed 3. Urban & Schwartzenberg, Baltimore and Munich, 1991, with permission.)

lar foramen in the petrosal ganglion. Their central processes pass through the jugular foramen and terminate in the nucleus solitarius. The somatic afferent component of the glossopharyngeal nerve is small and of little or no clinical importance. The cell bodies of these fibers are located in the jugular ganglion (superior ganglion of IX) and are believed to convey tactile information from the external ear canal. The central processes of these axons pass through the jugular foramen and terminate in the spinal nucleus of V.

Although the glossopharyngeal nerve is a mixed nerve composed of several functionally distinct fiber types, only its visceral afferent component has any clinical significance. Because it conveys tactile information from the pharyngeal mucosa, it serves as the afferent limb of the pharyngeal (gag) reflex. Details regarding the gag reflex are taken up in the next section, dealing with the vagus nerve. The vagus nerve mediates the motor component of the reflex.

Occasionally patients report symptoms referable to the glossopharyngeal nerve, most often a sense of numbness in the back of the throat. Unilateral numbness, together with an absent gag response to touching the pharyngeal wall on that side, would suggest disease involving the glossopharyngeal nerve. Bilateral lesions involving the glossopharyngeal nerve are rare, but when present, may be associated with an abrupt increase in blood pressure, which may last for up to 4 weeks before returning to premorbid levels.

VAGUS NERVE (X)

Functional Anatomy

The vagus nerve, like several other cranial nerves, is a mixed nerve composed of both sensory and motor fibers. The sensory fibers are mostly visceral in nature and transmit information from thoracic and abdominal visceral structures, chemoreceptors in the carotid body, and taste receptors on the epiglottis. The cell bodies of these visceral afferent fibers are located in the nodose ganglion, located immediately outside the jugular foramen (Fig. 17). The central processes of visceral afferent fibers of the vagus nerve pass through the jugular foramen and synapse in the nucleus solitarius. The vagus nerve is also believed to contain somatic afferent fibers, which mediate tactile sensation from the external ear canal. The cell bodies of somatic afferent fibers are located in the small jugular ganglion (superior ganglion of X), the source of a small number of axons that terminate in the spinal nucleus of V.

The motor component of the vagus nerve originates from two nuclei in the rostral medulla: the nucleus ambiguus and the dorsal motor nucleus of X. Axons arising from nerve cell bodies in the nucleus ambiguus

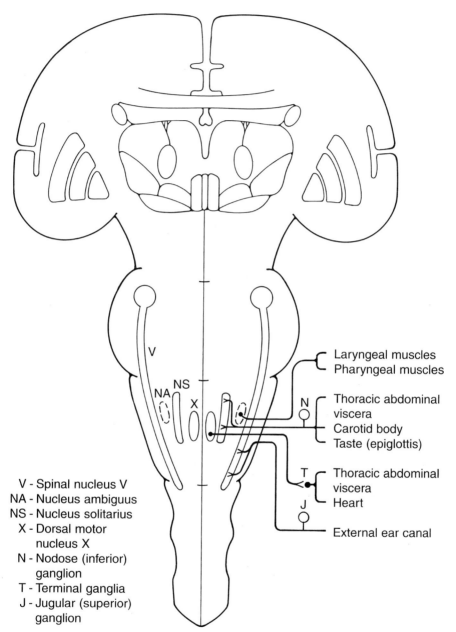

FIGURE 17. The central nuclei and peripheral ganglia associated with the vagus nerve (X). (Modified from Haines, DE: *Neuroanatomy: An Atlas of Structures, Sections, and Systems*, ed 3. Urban & Schwartzenberg, Baltimore and Munich, 1991, with permission.)

leave the cranium by way of the jugular foramen and distribute to the muscles of the soft palate, the pharyngeal constrictors, and the intrinsic and extrinsic muscles of the larynx. The dorsal motor nucleus of X contains preganglionic parasympathetic nerve cell bodies. The axons of these cells leave the cranium by way of the jugular foramen and distribute widely in the thorax and abdomen. In these regions, they make synaptic contact with postganglionic parasympathetic neurons, which in the thorax are associated with various plexuses such as the pulmonary and cardiac plexus. In the abdomen, they are in the wall of, or very near, the visceral structures (smooth muscle and glands) that they innervate.

Clinical Examinations

Lesions of the vagus nerve proximal to the branch point of nerve fibers innervating the pharyngeal muscles may produce difficulty with swallowing (dysphagia), which may be reported by the patient or which can be easily tested by having the patient drink a glass of water at examination. In addition, nasal escape or regurgitation may be present with phonation. To test for nasal escape (the escape of air through the nasal cavity while uttering plosive sounds), a cold mirror should be placed below the nostrils while the patient says "pa pa pa pa." Misting of the mirror with the utterance of plosive sounds indicates nasal escape and suggests a loss of innervation to the muscles of the soft palate.

Two easily performed tests of vagal function are observation of the movement of the uvula and soft palate with phonation and elicitation of the pharyngeal (gag) reflex. In the first test, the patient is asked to open the mouth wide while the tongue is kept relaxed in the floor of the mouth. The examiner first inspects the uvula and the free posterior margins of the soft palate. A tongue blade may be necessary to keep the tongue from blocking vision of the uvula and soft palate. In the normal individual, the uvula should be symmetric in shape and located essentially in the midline. Slight asymmetries in appearance or displacement from the midline are not necessarily indicative of vagal nerve lesions, however. Grossly apparent asymmetry of the soft palate or deviation of the uvula without phonation suggests a unilateral vagal nerve lesion. The test is completed by observing the movement of the uvula and soft palate when the patient says "Ah." The normal response is symmetric elevation of the soft palate without movement of the uvula in either direction. Unilateral lesions involving the vagus nerve are characterized by an inability to elevate the soft palate on the involved side, together with deviation of the uvula away from that side. Stated differently, patients with unilateral involvement of the vagus nerve demonstrate deviation of the uvula to the normal side with phonation. The observed response should be documented in the patient's record.

The pharyngeal (gag) reflex may also be used to evaluate the vagus nerve. The test is performed by gently touching the lateral pharyngeal wall near the tonsilar fossa with an orange stick or cotton-tipped applicator. The normal response is a strong contraction of the upper pharyngeal muscles (gagging). Both sides of the pharynx must be tested, because each is ipsilaterally innervated by afferent fibers carried in the glossopharyngeal nerve. Unilateral lesions involving the glossopharyngeal nerve will be characterized by a normal gag response to stimulation on the intact side and a loss of response to stimulation on the involved side. It should be noted that the gag reflex is sometimes absent in elderly patients who have no other evidence of neurologic impairment related to the glossopharyngeal or vagus nerves. A description of the response to stimulation of both sides should be noted in the patient's record.

Information obtained in the neurologic history, particularly the review of systems, may suggest involvement of the vagus nerve. For example, a change in voice quality in which the voice sounds hoarse (dysphonia) may indicate unilateral or bilateral lesions involving the vagus nerve. Diplophonia (the auditory perception of two pitch levels heard at the same time) with speaking may also be present in cases of unilateral lesions involving fibers that innervate the laryngeal muscles. Bilateral damage to the recurrent laryngeal branch of the vagus nerve results in denervation of the laryngeal muscles (laryngoplegia), which in turn results in adduction of the vocal folds. Patients with bilateral involvement of the vagus nerve have severe airway restriction evidenced by dyspnea, difficulty with coughing, and significant inspiratory stridor. These patients may require tracheostomy.

SPINAL ACCESSORY NERVE (XI)

Functional Anatomy

The spinal accessory nerve is a motor nerve that innervates the sternocleidomastoid and trapezius muscles. Although the spinal accessory nerve is considered a cranial nerve, its cells of origin are in upper cervical segments of the spinal cord. Specifically, nerve cells located in the dorsolateral part of the ventral horn (accessory process) at C-1 to C-4 give rise to axons that course laterally through the lateral funiculus to emerge from the spinal cord immediately dorsal to the denticulate ligament (Fig. 18). The axons course rostrally in the subarachnoid space and collect into a single bundle to enter the cranium through the foramen magnum. Within the cranium, the fibers course toward the jugular foramen, through which they pass to exit the skull together with the glossopharyngeal and vagus nerves. While in the cranium, they lie in close proximity to axons originating in the nucleus ambiguus that will be incorporated into the vagus nerve to innervate the muscles of the larynx and

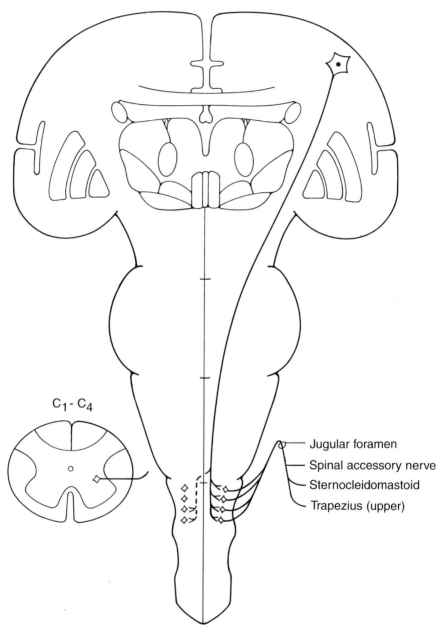

$C_1 - C_4$

Jugular foramen
Spinal accessory nerve
Sternocleidomastoid
Trapezius (upper)

FIGURE 18. The central and peripheral connections of the spinal accessory nerve (XI). (Modified from Haines, DE: *Neuroanatomy: An Atlas of Structures, Sections, and Systems*, ed 3. Urban & Schwartzenberg, Baltimore and Munich, 1991, with permission.)

pharynx. After passing out of the skull, the axons of the spinal accessory nerve course through the neck before dividing into branches that innervate the sternocleidomastoid and trapezius muscles.

Clinical Examinations

The spinal accessory nerve is tested by determining the strength of the sternocleidomastoid and trapezius muscles. Contraction of the sternocleidomastoid muscle bilaterally produces flexion of the head. Unilateral contraction causes turning of the face to the opposite side. The trapezius muscle is an upward rotator of the scapula and is therefore involved in shoulder elevation. Some authors have suggested that only the upper part of the trapezius muscle is innervated by the spinal accessory nerve, with the lower portions of the muscle receiving motor innervation by way of cervical spinal nerves. It also has been suggested that the sternocleidomastoid muscle is primarily innervated by cells located in the C-1 and C-2 segments of the spinal cord, whereas the upper trapezius muscle receives its motor innervation primarily from cells located in the C-3 and C-4 segments.

Clinical assessment of the spinal accessory nerve should begin with inspection of the neck and shoulders and palpation of the two muscles. Asymmetry of the neck by visual inspection or with a deep, forced inspiration may suggest unilateral lesions. Wasting of the upper trapezius muscle or a particularly prominent acromion process may also be seen with unilateral lesions. Slight winging of the scapula may also be evident. At rest, the face will typically not be turned to one side or the other.

It is important for the examiner to palpate the sternocleidomastoid and trapezius muscles at rest, paying particular attention to their bulk and contour. The examiner may stand in front of or behind the patient to palpate both sternocleidomastoid muscles simultaneously, being sure to examine the relatively free anterior margins and the bulk of the muscle from origin to insertion. The patient should then be asked to turn the face to one side while the examiner palpates the contralateral sternocleidomastoid muscle. The examiner then pushes on the patient's maxilla in an attempt to bring the face to the forward position while still palpating the contralateral sternocleidomastoid muscle. The process should be repeated, asking the patient to turn the face in the other direction.

Strength is graded on a five-point scale:

0—no contraction
1—trace contraction
2—poor contraction
3—fair contraction
4—good contraction
5—normal contraction

(*Note:* A more complete description of muscle testing and grading appears in Chapter 5, pages 127 to 134.) Strength of contraction is recorded as a fraction. For example, 5/5 suggests normal strength for that muscle, whereas 1/5 would indicate a barely palpable contraction.

To test the trapezius muscle, the examiner asks the patient to elevate or shrug the shoulders. The examiner then attempts to push down on the shoulders simultaneously, looking for both differences in the strength of the patient between the two sides and the amount of force the patient can muster to overcome the examiner's effort to force the shoulders down. Muscle strength grading is the same as that described above.

Another simple test for trapezius muscle function is for the examiner to ask the patient to reach forward as far as possible and place the palms together. In cases of unilateral weakness of the trapezius muscle, the fingers on the involved side may extend slightly farther forward than those on the uninvolved side, because the trapezius muscle is also involved in scapular retraction. When the patient reaches forward, the scapulae will protract to increase range of reach. Some tension on the normal side will restrict protraction slightly, thus reducing by a small amount the forward reach on that side so that the fingers on the involved side will extend slightly farther forward.

Clinical evidence suggests that corticospinal projections that influence sternocleidomastoid lower motor neurons are ipsilateral in distribution, whereas projections to trapezius lower motor neurons may be either ipsilateral or contralateral. This idea is based in part on the observation that hemiplegic patients frequently present with paresis of the ipsilateral sternocleidomastoid and contralateral trapezius muscles.

Some authors have noted that corticospinal projections to lower motor neurons innervating the sternocleidomastoid and trapezius muscles are separated in the brainstem. It has been suggested that projections that influence the sternocleidomastoid muscle course through the brainstem tegmentum, whereas those that influence the trapezius muscle are located more ventrally, in close association with the fibers of the pyramidal system. This arrangement of fibers may explain why some patients with ventral pontine lesions demonstrate paresis involving the trapezius muscle but sparing the sternocleidomastoid muscle. A similar clinical picture may be seen in patients with middle to low cervical lesions involving only the C-3 and C-4 segments and below. Such patients demonstrate weakness of the trapezius muscle but little or no involvement of the sternocleidomastoid muscle. This observation strengthens the notion that the sternocleidomastoid and trapezius muscles receive motor innervation from different segments of the spinal cord.

HYPOGLOSSAL NERVE (XII)

Functional Anatomy

The hypoglossal nerve provides motor innervation to the intrinsic and extrinsic muscles of the tongue. The nerve originates from lower motor neurons located near the midline in the rostral part of the medulla oblongata (Fig. 19). The axons course ventrolaterally through the brainstem tegmentum and lie between the inferior olivary nucleus and the medullary pyramid. They emerge from the brainstem along a shallow sulcus that separates these two grossly visible structures. Once outside the brainstem, the axons travel toward the hypoglossal canal, by which they exit the skull. For clinical purposes, the most important muscles innervated by the hypoglossal nerve are the intrinsic tongue muscles and the genioglossus muscle, which causes protrusion of the tongue.

Clinical Examination

Testing hypoglossal nerve function begins with careful observation of the tongue resting in the floor of the mouth. The examiner should carefully examine the mass and contour of the tongue and note any movements such as fasciculation or fibrillations. Unilateral lesions of the hypoglossal nerve may produce atrophy on the ipsilateral side, frequently associated with fibrillations — small, contraction-like movements that are evident when the tongue is at rest. Fibrillations may not be evident when the tongue is protruded.

Next, the patient should be asked to protrude the tongue in the midline. The examiner should instruct the patient to "Stick your tongue out" and observe whether the tongue remains in the midline or deviates to one side or the other. In patients with unilateral involvement of the hypoglossal nerve, the tongue may deviate toward the side of involvement. Deviation to the side of the lesion is a result of the failure of the genioglossus muscle on that side to pull the tongue fully out of the mouth. The protruded tongue may also appear wrinkled and slightly elevated on the involved side because of the pull of the muscles on the uninvolved side.

The patient should then be asked to push the tongue into the cheek on one side. The examiner should press on the cheek in an attempt to force the tongue out of the cheek. The procedure should then be repeated on the other side. Unilateral hypoglossal nerve damage will be characterized by a relative ease in pushing the tongue out of the cheek on the uninvolved side. This is an important component of the test because some patients with only minor weakness may be able to protrude

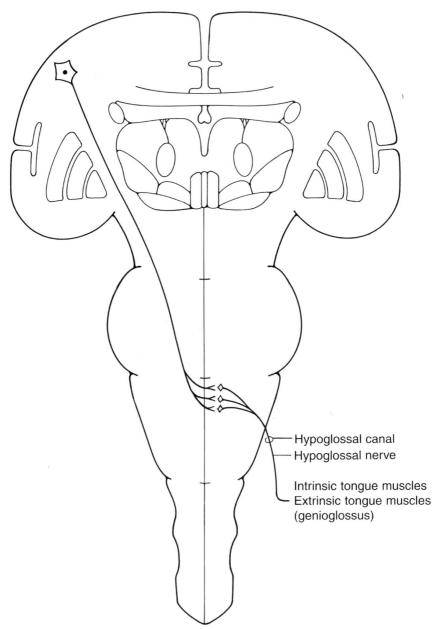

FIGURE 19. The central and peripheral connections of the hypoglossal nerve (XII). (Modified from Haines, DE: *Neuroanatomy: An Atlas of Structures, Sections, and Systems*, ed 3. Urban & Schwartzenberg, Baltimore and Munich, 1991, with permission.)

the tongue in the midline but will be unable to keep the tongue forced into the cheek.

Patients with hypoglossal nerve lesions typically have difficulty with uttering lingual sounds. A simple test is to ask the patient to say "la la la," "tee, tee, tee," or "dee, dee, dee." These sounds will be poorly performed because normal enunciation requires pushing the tongue against the hard palate. In a similar way, patients with lesions involving the hypoglossal nerve may also report difficulty with manipulation of food in the mouth and with swallowing (dysphagia). Patients with bilateral lesions of the hypoglossal nerve may have difficulty with respiration because the tongue tends to fall backward into the oropharynx.

Corticobulbar projections to the hypoglossal nucleus are contralateral in distribution. Lesions involving these upper motor neuron projections, such as those that may be seen in the hemiplegic patient, may be characterized by difficulty with lingual sounds, weakness of lateral tongue movements to the contralateral side, and deviation of the tongue to the contralateral (hemiplegic) side with protrusion. Patients with upper motor neuron lesions may also have difficulty with rapid protrusion-retraction movements of the tongue, but they generally do not demonstrate atrophy or fibrillations, because corticobulbar projections to the intrinsic muscles of the tongue are thought to be bilateral.

The results obtained with testing should be thoroughly documented to include the presence or absence of atrophy, fasciculation, or fibrillations; deviation to the side with protrusion; weakness with lateral movements; and difficulty with lingual sounds, food manipulation, swallowing, or respiration.

CHAPTER 5

MOTOR SYSTEMS (INCLUDING COORDINATION)

The motor systems are composed of functionally organized groups of neurons that regulate muscle activity necessary for the maintenance of posture and the purposeful and coordinated perturbations of posture we refer to as movement. Although an essential purpose of these neuronal systems in animals and humans is to help ensure survival, in humans they function to help individuals achieve other, more varied and desirable goals. From a clinical perspective, the motor systems make it possible for individuals to express their wants, needs, feelings, experiences, and general state of health and well-being. Motor system dysfunction not only can make it difficult for people to carry out activities of daily living efficiently and effectively but, in more extreme cases, may deprive them of the ability to satisfy basic needs or even to communicate their wants and needs to others. The clinician therefore must be able to recognize motor disturbances, understand their meaning and significance, and take corrective measures when possible or necessary.

To organize our approach to the examination of the motor systems, we have divided the motor systems into peripheral and central components. The peripheral components consist of alpha and gamma motor neurons, their axons, the skeletal muscles they innervate, and the neuromuscular junction. The central components consist of functionally organized groups of neurons in the forebrain, brainstem, and cerebellum, which are known to influence the activity of alpha and gamma motor neurons.

The following brief summary of the organization of the peripheral and central components of the motor systems will acquaint or reacquaint the reader with fundamental concepts that form the basis for specific tests of motor function and will help the clinician to interpret the results of these tests.

PERIPHERAL COMPONENTS

The peripheral components of the motor systems are composed of muscles of various types and the neurons that innervate them. Physiologically and functionally, we can identify two distinct types of muscles: extrafusal muscles and intrafusal muscles. *Extrafusal muscles* cross one or more joints and therefore are directly involved in the control of posture and the production of movement. Extrafusal muscles are innervated by alpha motor neurons, so named because they transmit nerve impulses at velocities that define the alpha range (80 to 120 meters per second). *Intrafusal muscles* are small, striated muscles located in the polar regions of the muscle spindle. Contraction of intrafusal muscle fibers increases tension in the muscle spindle but does not result in movement. Muscle spindles are innervated by gamma motor neurons, so named because they transmit nerve impulses more slowly, at velocities that define the gamma range (15 to 30 meters per second).

An important concept regarding the peripheral components of the motor system is the *motor unit*, defined as consisting of an alpha motor neuron, its axon and collateral branches, and all of the skeletal muscle fibers it innervates. Motor units in muscles used for fine, skilled movements such as speech, eye control, or manipulation tasks with the hands tend to be small, meaning that the ratio of alpha motor neurons to the number of skeletal muscle fibers they innervate is low. In contrast, motor units in muscles used predominantly for postural and locomotor activities, such as the paraspinal and limb-girdle muscles, tend to be considerably larger, with a single alpha motor neuron providing motor innervation to many skeletal muscle fibers.

Alpha motor neurons are frequently referred to as *lower motor neurons*; with their axons and collateral branches, they constitute the final common pathway by which nerve impulses reach skeletal muscles to cause them to contract. The final common pathway, therefore, is the final link in the chain of neurons that control posture and movement.

CENTRAL COMPONENTS

The central components of the motor systems are functionally more numerous and organizationally more complicated than are the peripheral components. For our purposes, two distinct types of central nervous system neurons that influence motor behavior can be described: upper motor neurons and neurons composing functional systems that influence upper motor neurons. With regard to the latter, this discussion will be limited to the neurons and neuronal pathways commonly associated with the cerebellum and basal nuclei.

Upper Motor Neurons (Cortical)

Clinically, the term *upper motor neuron* is generally used to refer to nerve cells located in the primary motor regions of the cerebral cortex. These cells are located in the posterior part of the frontal lobe (areas 4, 6, and 8) and in the anterior part of the parietal lobe (areas 3, 1, 2, and 5). In the neurologic examination, we frequently divide cortical upper motor neurons into two groups: those that influence alpha and gamma motor neurons located in cranial nerve motor nuclei and those that influence alpha and gamma motor neurons located in the ventral horn of the spinal cord. Axons of the former compose the corticonuclear (corticobulbar) tracts, which were considered in Chapter 4 in connection with the examination of cranial nerve function. Axons of the latter compose the corticospinal system, which courses through the brainstem to influence lower motor neurons in the spinal cord. The motor systems examination focuses primarily on motor functions mediated by spinal motor neurons.

Corticospinal upper motor neurons are organized somatotopically in the primary motor cortices of the posterior frontal and anterior parietal lobes. Corticospinal neurons that influence lower motor neurons located at lumbar and sacral spinal levels are found along the medial surface of the hemisphere, in the sagittal sulcus, whereas those that affect lower motor neurons of cervical and upper thoracic levels are located on the dorsal and dorsolateral surfaces of the hemisphere. The axons of these cells course through the subcortical white matter (corona radiata) immediately deep to the cortical areas from which they arise (Fig. 20). At the level of the thalamus, they lie in the posterior limb of the internal capsule; at the level of the midbrain, they lie in the middle portion of the cerebral peduncle. Corticospinal fibers retain their somatotopic organization in both the internal capsule and the cerebral peduncle. The fibers pass through the pontine nuclei, and at the level of the medulla oblongata, they lie on its ventral surface, forming the medullary pyramid. The majority of these axons cross the midline in the pyramidal decussation. In the spinal cord, corticospinal axons that crossed the midline in the pyramidal decussation constitute the lateral corticospinal tract, and those that remained uncrossed form the anterior (ventral) corticospinal tract. Within the spinal gray matter, these axons make either direct or indirect synaptic contact with the dendrites of alpha motor neurons and, to a lesser degree, with those of gamma motor neurons.

Historically, corticospinal axons have frequently been referred to as part of the *pyramidal system*, a name reflecting the fact that the axons are located within the medullary pyramid. The term *corticospinal system* is sometimes also used to refer to these fibers. For the sake of precision and to avoid needless confusion, however, the term *corticospinal tract* should be used to refer specifically to the spinal part of this cortically originating descending motor system.

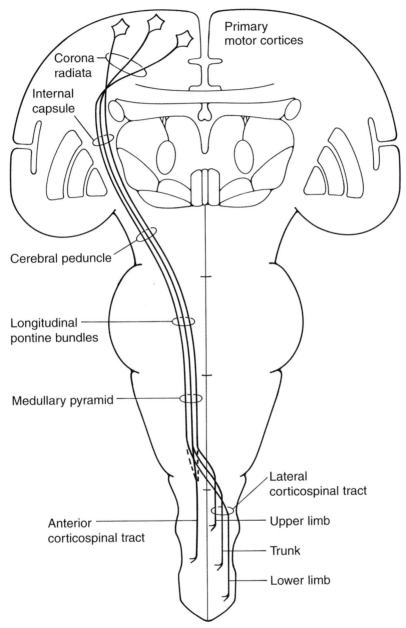

FIGURE 20. The corticospinal (pyramidal) system. (Modified from Haines, DE: *Neuroanatomy: An Atlas of Structures, Sections, and Systems*, ed 3. Urban & Schwartzenberg, Baltimore and Munich, 1991, with permission.)

A few clinically important anatomic facts about this system are worth highlighting at this time. First, about 85 to 90 percent of the approximately 1 million axons that form each medullary pyramid decussate at caudal medullary levels to achieve a position in the contralateral half of the spinal cord. These axons occupy a position in the dorsal part of the lateral funiculus and are organized somatotopically so that those axons that will terminate at rostral spinal levels are located medial to those that will terminate at more caudal levels (see Fig. 20). Collectively, these axons constitute the lateral corticospinal tract, which extends the full length of the spinal cord. Axons that do not cross the midline in the pyramidal decussation maintain their ventral position within the spinal cord and are located in the ventral funiculus of the spinal cord, where they constitute the anterior (ventral) corticospinal tract. Axons of the anterior corticospinal tract also extend the full length of the spinal cord but do not seem to be somatotopically organized within the ventral funiculus.

The relative position of the lateral and anterior corticospinal tracts within the spinal white matter suggests that they may preferentially influence specific lower motor neuron pools within the ventral horn. Clinical as well as anatomic evidence indicates that lateral corticospinal tract axons influence predominantly limb-related lower motor neurons, whereas anterior corticospinal tract axons seem to exert their effects on neurons innervating axial muscle groups. Moreover, lateral corticospinal tract axons that terminate at spinal levels forming the brachial plexus seem to exert a greater influence on lower motor neurons that innervate the finger flexors and wrist extensors than on other functionally related groups of lower motor neurons.

Second, axons composing the lateral corticospinal tract are not equally distributed to all levels of the spinal cord. Estimates indicate that approximately 55 percent of the axons forming the lateral corticospinal tract terminate at spinal levels contributing to the brachial plexus (C-5 through T-1), with an additional 25 percent ending in spinal segments of origin of the lumbosacral plexus (L-2 through S-2). Lateral corticospinal tract axons terminate within the spinal gray matter on the ipsilateral side.

In contrast, the axons of the anterior corticospinal tract seem to be distributed fairly evenly to all spinal segments. Moreover, unlike lateral corticospinal axons, as many as 50 percent of the axons of the anterior corticospinal tract may recross the midline in the anterior white commissure of the spinal cord to make synaptic contact with alpha motor neurons in the medial portion of the ventral horn on the contralateral side. This observation suggests that axial muscles, which are innervated by lower motor neurons in the medial portion of the ventral horn, receive synaptic input from both cerebral hemispheres, whereas limb muscles (particularly distal limb muscles) are influenced exclusively by the contralateral cerebral cortex.

A third clinically important fact regarding corticospinal axons concerns those that decussate at the level of the caudal medulla in the pyramidal decussation. Axons that terminate at more rostral levels of the spinal cord decussate most rostrally in the pyramidal decussation, while those destined for more caudal spinal levels cross more caudally in the pyramidal decussation (see Fig. 20). This observation may be valuable when interpreting motor findings produced by small, localized lesions in the ventral part of the caudal medulla.

Upper Motor Neurons (Brainstem)

In addition to the cerebral cortex, certain brainstem nuclei also contain upper motor neurons. Chief among these nuclei are the red nucleus, the vestibular nuclei, the nuclei of the superior colliculus, and nuclei of the mesencephalic tegmentum.

Red Nucleus

The red nucleus is the origin of axons that cross the midline at caudal mesencephalic levels and lie in the lateral part of the brainstem reticular formation. In the spinal cord, these axons lie intermingled with those of the lateral corticospinal tract and, like lateral corticospinal tract axons, terminate in motor nuclei located largely in the lateral part of the ventral horn (Fig. 21). The majority of the axons of the rubrospinal tract end at the level of the cervical enlargement, although the tract has been shown to extend caudally to upper sacral levels. Clinical evidence suggests that the red nucleus influences upper limb flexor muscle groups predominantly, although effects on other upper limb muscle groups cannot be ruled out. The position of rubrospinal axons within the spinal cord at more caudal levels would suggest that they influence flexor muscle groups of the lower limb more than extensor muscles. It is unlikely that rubrospinal tract axons exert any significant influence on lower motor neurons that innervate axial muscles.

Vestibular Nuclei

The vestibular nuclei are the origin of two descending tracts that influence spinal lower motor neurons. The lateral vestibulospinal tract originates from the lateral vestibular nucleus (Deiter's nucleus) and lies in the ventral part of the ipsilateral lateral funiculus (see Fig. 21). The tract extends the full length of the spinal cord, suggesting that it influences motor neurons innervating both upper and lower limb muscles. The location of these axons within the spinal white matter suggests further that their influence is exerted predominantly on extensor muscle groups of the upper and lower limbs. The inferior and medial vestibular nuclei are the ori-

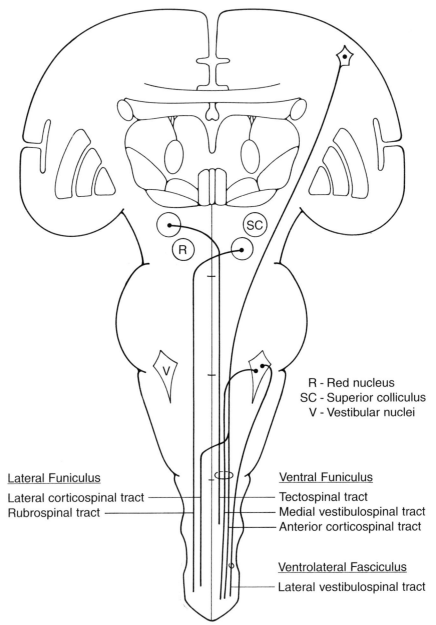

R - Red nucleus
SC - Superior colliculus
V - Vestibular nuclei

Lateral Funiculus

Lateral corticospinal tract
Rubrospinal tract

Ventral Funiculus

Tectospinal tract
Medial vestibulospinal tract
Anterior corticospinal tract

Ventrolateral Fasciculus

Lateral vestibulospinal tract

FIGURE 21. The origin, course, and location within the spinal cord of major upper motor neuron pathways. (Modified from Haines, DE: *Neuroanatomy: An Atlas of Structures, Sections, and Systems*, ed 3. Urban & Schwartzenberg, Baltimore and Munich, 1991, with permission.)

gin of axons that lie medially in the caudal brainstem, intermixed with the axons of the medial longitudinal fasciculus. In the spinal cord, these axons form the medial vestibulospinal tract and are found in the ventral funiculus of the spinal cord. The medial vestibulospinal tract contains axons originating from both the ipsilateral and contralateral vestibular nuclei. The position of these axons in the ventral funiculus of the spinal cord suggests that they preferentially influence axial muscle groups, particularly extensor muscles of the neck and trunk. Clinical and experimental evidence supports the idea that the vestibulospinal pathways exert excitatory effects on extensor muscles of the limbs, particularly limb-girdle muscles, and on extensor muscles of the neck and trunk.

Nuclei of the Superior Colliculus

The superior colliculus is the origin of axons that cross the midline at midmesencephalic levels to occupy a position immediately ventral to the medial longitudinal fasciculus. Within the spinal cord, tectospinal axons are located in the ventral funiculus and seem to extend caudally only to cervical and upper thoracic levels (see Fig. 21). Clinical evidence suggests that the tectobulbar component of this descending fiber system is involved in the control of extraocular muscles, and the tectospinal component influences cervical muscles involved in controlling the position of the head. This pathway seems to be involved in linking extraocular movements with head movements to allow control of the field of vision.

Other nuclei located in the tegmentum of the midbrain (that is, dorsal and ventral tegmental nuclei) are the origin of descending projections that influence lower motor neurons in the brainstem and spinal cord. The dorsal tegmental nuclei may be thought of as the origin of tegmentobulbar pathways, and the ventral nuclei as the origin of the tegmentospinal pathways. The effect of nerve impulse conduction along these pathways is unclear; it may be important in regulating the excitability of both alpha and gamma motor neurons and related interneurons.

Because the axons of upper motor neurons located in the brainstem are *not* found in the medullary pyramid, they are properly referred to as *extrapyramidal pathways*, a term that has given rise to the notion of an extrapyramidal system or systems. Unfortunately, the precise function of these descending motor pathways is still unclear. Unfortunate also is the frequent use of the term "extrapyramidal disease" to refer to disease processes involving particular telencephalic and diencephalic nuclei, rather than to refer more correctly to diseases involving brainstem nuclei that are the origin of descending motor pathways *not* located in the medullary pyramid. I advocate the abandonment of the terms "extrapyramidal systems" and "extrapyramidal diseases," which are no longer adequate descriptions. The persistent misuse of these terms, particularly as we develop a better understanding of the organization and function of the nervous system, leads to more confusion than clarity and, in fact, may hinder efforts to further our understanding.

Upper motor neurons located in both the cerebral cortex and the brainstem are a major source of synaptic input to lower motor neurons. Some of the neurons in the cerebral cortex, particularly those that influence distal limb function, make direct synaptic contact with alpha motor neurons, whereas others exert indirect effects by way of local *interneurons*. Brainstem upper motor neurons are thought to influence lower motor neurons largely, if not exclusively, through interneuronal connections. Interneurons serve two important functions related to the motor systems and motor behavior. First, normal motor behavior is the product of many muscles and muscle groups (agonists, antagonists, and synergists) acting together to achieve a purposeful goal. Interneuronal connections linking lower motor neuron pools at different levels of the neuraxis are the anatomic substrate on which multisegmental motor behaviors are built. Second, normal motor behavior requires that some muscles relax while others contract. Inhibition of lower motor neurons is therefore just as important as excitation for normal motor behavior. These important inhibitory functions are considered to be mediated by specific groups of local interneurons.

Finally, we must consider several specialized regions of the brain, which, by virtue of their fiber connections, influence the activity of the upper motor neurons just described. Three functionally and clinically distinct sources of input to upper motor neurons are considered:

1. The association cortex
2. The basal nuclei
3. The cerebellum

Although volumes could be written about the importance of each of these areas to motor behavior, only a brief review is presented here. This brief synopsis is intended to make the tests of motor function described later in the chapter and their interpretation seem reasonable and appropriate.

Association Cortex

The cerebral cortex is a functionally diverse collection of nerve cells. One way of ordering our thinking is to distinguish between primary cortical areas (sensory and motor) and association areas of the cortex. *Primary sensory cortices* receive input from specific thalamic nuclei, or, in the case of smell, from the olfactory bulb. *Primary motor cortices*, by definition, contain neurons that contribute axons to the corticospinal and corticobulbar (corticonuclear) tracts. The remaining areas of the cerebral cortex are referred to as *association cortices*. Many authors further divide the association cortices into sensory association cortex and motor association cortex.

The primary sensory cortices project heavily to related sensory association cortices, where some interpretation of the sensory experience takes place. Sensory association cortices, in turn, project to other association cortices within the same hemisphere and, through the corpus callosum and other commissural connections, to association cortices in the contralateral hemisphere. Many sensory association areas project in turn to the primary motor and motor association cortices, thereby providing cortical upper motor neurons with information transmitted to and processed by brain areas associated with the sensory systems.

The prefrontal areas of the frontal lobe are a rich source of input to the primary motor cortices, particularly to those areas lying anterior to the central sulcus. The ability of association cortices to influence cortical upper motor neurons is thought to be important not only in the control of simple voluntary movements but also in the regulation and expression of emotionally charged motor behaviors. Thus, upper motor neurons located in the primary motor cortices can be influenced by a wide variety of cortical areas, each of which may be involved in very different aspects of brain function. Damage to association areas of the cerebral cortex or to the axons that interconnect these areas with the motor cortex typically presents as apraxias and agnosias. Other signs and symptoms not associated with motor function may also be produced by lesions that affect the motor and sensory association cortices.

Basal Nuclei

The *basal nuclei* are a group of subcortical structures located deep within each cerebral hemisphere. They consist of the striatum (caudate and putamen), the globus pallidus, and the amygdaloid nucleus. Input to the basal nuclei originates largely from the cerebral cortex and is directed mainly to the striatum. The striatum also receives synaptic input from the substantia nigra. Striatal efferent neurons terminate largely in the globus pallidus. The globus pallidus is the major output nucleus of the basal nuclei and is the origin of fibers that influence upper motor neurons in both the brainstem (red nucleus and dorsal and ventral tegmental nuclei) and cerebral cortex (corticospinal and corticobulbar neurons). Influences exerted on cortical upper motor neurons are mediated by way of projections through the ventral anterior and ventral lateral nuclei of the thalamus. The globus pallidus is strongly influenced by neurons located in the subthalamic nucleus. Although the exact role of the basal nuclei and their associated nuclei in the control of posture and movement remains unclear, specific deficits associated with disease or injury involving several of these nuclei are well characterized.

An oversimplified, although perhaps useful, idea regarding the function of the basal nuclei is to consider them important in determining *which* upper motor neurons need to be activated (or inhibited) to produce a desired motor behavior. This idea is based on clinical observations suggesting that motor deficits associated with diseases involving the basal nuclei are characterized by the inappropriate recruitment of motor units (too many or too few) for the intended behavioral task. In some cases, movements are difficult to initiate, and in others, unintended or unneeded movements are present. Not infrequently, both types of problems are evident in the same patient.

Cerebellum

The *cerebellum* receives input from the vestibular apparatus, muscle spindles located throughout the body, the inferior olivary nuclei, and the cerebral cortex by way of the pontine nuclei. Like the basal nuclei, the output of the cerebellum is directed toward upper motor neurons in the brainstem and cerebral cortex. Brainstem upper motor neurons influenced by the cerebellum are located chiefly in the red nucleus and the vestibular nuclei. Cortical upper motor neurons are those that give rise to the corticospinal and corticobulbar tracts. Cerebellar influences on cortical upper motor neurons, like those of the basal nuclei, are mediated by way of projections through the ventral lateral nucleus of the thalamus. Clinical observations suggest that the cerebellum is important in determining *when* upper motor neurons need to be activated (or inhibited) to produce a desired movement. Motor deficits associated with diseases of the cerebellum are characterized by an inappropriate sequencing in the activation and deactivation of upper motor neurons and, consequently, of lower motor neurons. Patients with cerebellar disease appear to have difficulty adjusting the amplitude, direction, and velocity of their intended movements.

In summary, lower motor neurons and their axons represent the final common pathway that leads to muscle contraction. Lower motor neurons are influenced by upper motor neurons located in both the cerebral cortex and brainstem. Upper motor neuron influences are mediated largely by way of local interneurons, which can exert either excitatory or inhibitory effects on lower motor neuron pools. Upper motor neurons, in turn, are influenced by a wide range of brain areas, including association areas of the cerebral cortex, the basal nuclei, and the cerebellum. Ultimately, the function of the motor systems is to excite or inhibit selected lower motor neuron pools required to carry out a particular motor behavior, and to do so in the proper sequence. The signs and symptoms produced by lesions affecting particular components of the motor system reflect an inability to properly carry out these two important physiologic processes. The next section considers specific clinical tests to evaluate various aspects of motor function.

CLINICAL EXAMINATIONS

The examination of motor function, although formally conducted after an evaluation of mental status and the cranial nerves, actually begins early in the patient encounter. Careful observation of the patient sitting in the waiting room, moving into the examining room, or lying in the hospital bed can provide important information about the functional integrity of the motor systems. The alert and attentive clinician, like Sherlock Holmes, not only sees what everyone else sees but also recognizes the significance of observations that inexperienced or inattentive observers may only record.

Among those aspects of motor behavior that should be observed early in the patient encounter are posture, speech pattern, and movement. With regard to posture, it is useful to observe the resting position of the limbs, trunk, head, eyes, and eyelids. Motor behaviors that are easily observed but frequently overlooked include speech prosody and volume, blink frequency, ocular movements, and breathing. Some patients demonstrate a paucity of movement while others appear to be constantly in motion. Certain motor behaviors will be detected as frankly abnormal, but others may be masked or incorporated into seemingly appropriate acts, giving the impression of normality. With experience, the alert clinician can recognize and identify even the most subtle abnormalities of motor behavior.

A judgment should be made as to whether the patient's movements are normal and appropriate or abnormal in some definable way. Abnormal movements may occur because of weakness involving particular muscles or muscle groups. In such cases, the observed movements may reflect the substitution of normal or less involved muscles for weak or paralyzed muscles. In other cases, unintended muscle contractions or inappropriate and unwanted movements may be seen. Some types of abnormal movements are diagnostic, and others can produce a high index of suspicion regarding a particular neurologic disease.

The motor examination should begin with the formal processes of inspection, palpation, and when indicated, percussion. Inspection should focus on the *bulk, contour,* and *symmetry* of individual muscles and muscle groups. The clinician should look for atrophy or hypertrophy and carefully note its distribution. The distribution of atrophic muscles frequently helps to localize the site of the atrophy-producing lesion. Two types of atrophy are generally recognized: disuse atrophy and denervation atrophy. *Disuse atrophy* can be seen in patients entirely free from neurologic disease who have been immobilized for some length of time. It can also be seen in patients with upper motor neuron lesions who are unable to use a particular muscle group or part of the body for everyday activities. In contrast, *denervation atrophy* is usually the result of damage to lower motor neurons or their axons, which interrupts conduction of nerve impulses to skeletal muscles. Over time, complete interruption results in a profound degree of atrophy and a flaccid paralysis (an inability to produce muscle contraction in response to voluntary effort or reflex stimulation).

Muscle tone and muscle stretch reflexes are frequently preserved in disuse atrophy but are usually reduced or lost in denervation atrophy. Trophic changes involving the skin and nails may be seen with denervation atrophy but not with disuse atrophy. In addition, the degree of muscle atrophy is generally greater in muscles that are denervated than in those that are normally innervated but simply are not being used for one reason or another.

Quantitative assessment of the degree of atrophy is easily accomplished by using a tape measure. Girth measurements may be a particularly useful way of measuring disease progression or regression over time or in response to therapeutic intervention. When measuring girth, it is important to carefully document the exact site from which the measurements are taken. Bony prominences are particularly good landmarks to use for this purpose.

Palpation is an important part of the motor examination. The clinician should note the consistency of the muscle in the resting condition and the presence of trigger points or contractures. Reports of tenderness and pain should be documented, with a description of their location, character, and duration. If pain is reported, the clinician should inquire about activities or factors that make it better or worse. Inquiries concerning weakness, clumsiness, stiffness, or difficulties with activities of daily living such as bathing, dressing, eating, walking, or speaking are essential and provide valuable information about the integrity of the motor systems. Such inquiries will also help to identify specific aspects of motor function that may require a more detailed evaluation.

A number of neurologic disorders are characterized by abnormalities of muscle control. Some are of sufficient magnitude to alter posture in grossly visible ways or produce unwanted or abnormal movement; others are evidenced only by isolated muscle cell contractions or activity involving a single motor unit, or perhaps several. *Fibrillations* are spontaneous, independent contractions of individual muscle fibers that are not visible through the skin. They generally become evident 8 to 12 days after denervation of a muscle and are detected by electromyography. Occasionally, fibrillations may be seen in the tongue when it is resting quietly in the floor of the mouth. Fibrillations involving the tongue cannot be seen when the tongue is protruded.

Fasciculations are spontaneous visible or palpable contractions of the muscle fibers associated with a single lower motor neuron. Fasciculations represent the spontaneous firing of individual motor units. Fasciculations can occur in normal individuals but are more commonly a sign of pathology. They are frequently seen in patients with diseases involving the lower motor neuron, such as amyotrophic lateral sclerosis. Percussion of a muscle may produce fasciculations in susceptible individuals. They may not be visible in obese patients or in deeply located muscles. Fibrillations and fasciculations do not produce changes in posture or abnormal movements of body parts.

Involuntary movements and inappropriate postures are not uncommon in patients with motor system disease. Table 9 presents a brief description of some of the more significant and frequently encountered motor abnormalities. Some are present continuously and have a sustained character (e.g., dystonia); some may be more rhythmic or oscillatory in nature (e.g., nystagmus). Other types are episodic or intermittent in appearance (e.g., myoclonus or tics) and can be extremely violent (ballismus). Involuntary movements may be evident when the patient is at rest (e.g., torticollis or rest tremor) or may appear only with the onset of movement (intention or action tremor).

Muscle Tone

An important function of the nervous system is the regulation of muscle tone. *Muscle tone* can be defined as the degree or strength of contraction that characterizes *normally innervated, resting* skeletal muscle. Muscle tone is produced by the ongoing activation of motor units, sufficient in number to provide a certain degree of muscle tension without producing movement. Normal muscle tone is a prerequisite for normal posture and movement. It follows, therefore, that patients with abnormal muscle tone will also demonstrate disordered posture and movement.

Muscle spindles play a major role in the regulation of muscle tone. They are essentially stretch receptors located within skeletal muscles, which monitor both the length of the muscle and the speed at which changes in length occur. Muscle spindles transmit nerve impulses to the central nervous system by way of type Ia and type II afferent fibers. Impulse transmission along spindle afferent fibers leads to excitation of the alpha motor neurons that innervate the skeletal muscle in which the stretched spindle is located.

The sensitivity of the muscle spindle to stretch is controlled by gamma motor neurons, which innervate the small intrafusal muscles located in the polar regions of the spindle. Increased gamma motor neuron activity leads to increased spindle sensitivity; decreased activity produces a decrease in spindle sensitivity. Clinically, hypersensitive muscle

TABLE 9 *Descriptive Characteristics of Selected Motor Disturbances*

Asterixis	A motor disturbance, most evident in the wrist, characterized by intermittent relaxation of extensor muscles when used to support the outstretched hands against gravity. The hand appears to flap in a waving or tremor-like motion. Frequently seen in patients suffering from liver failure.
Athetosis	An involuntary, ceaseless series of muscle contractions producing slow, sinuous, writhing movements, especially severe in the hands. Seen in some patients with cerebral palsy or hemiplegia.
Ballismus	Violent, spontaneous, and uncontrollable flinging or flailing movements of axial and limb-girdle muscles occurring as a result of lesions involving the subthalamic nucleus. Usually unilateral and very exhausting for the patient.
Blepharospasm	Tonic spasms of the orbicularis oculi muscle producing more or less complete closure of the eye. May occur in normal individuals or in patients with lesions of the eye or the trigeminal nerve.
Chorea	Involuntary, rapid, flowing movements manifested as random events present at rest. The movements are irregular and lack apparent purpose. They are frequently followed immediately by some voluntary motor behavior designed to mask the involuntary component, to make it appear to be part of a more purposeful, complex motor activity. Choreatic movements subside with sleep.
Cramp	An often painful muscle spasm typically seen in muscles used frequently or for prolonged periods of time (feet, calves, hands). May occur while resting or asleep but usually seen after strenuous activity (e.g., writer's cramp). Occurs in normal individuals but with greater frequency in patients with neurologic disease. Cramps are generally relieved by stretching.
Dysdiadochokinesia	An inability to alternately contract and relax agonist and antagonist muscles or muscle groups.
Dysmetria	An inability to control muscle action required to move a body part smoothly in a specific direction or along a particular course. Patients appear to have difficulty in regulating the direction and amplitude of voluntary movements.
Dystonia	Irregular, involuntary contractions of muscles of the head, limbs, or trunk, producing contortions or abnormal postures. More severe and sustained than cramps or simple muscle spasms.
Myoclonus	Involuntary, lightning-like muscle contractions appearing as single or repetitive jerks. Most commonly involves limb muscles but may also affect the muscles of the palate (palatal myoclonus). Contractions may be spontaneous or evoked by loud noises or visual or tactile stimuli. Myoclonus is seen in association with lesions of the central nervous system.
Myokymia	Brief, spontaneous, tetanic contractions of motor units, slower and more prolonged than fasciculations. Usually benign and associated with overuse but may be seen in patients with multiple sclerosis or other demyelinating diseases.

TABLE 9 *Descriptive Characteristics of Selected Motor Disturbances (Continued)*

Myotonia	A condition characterized by increased muscular irritability and contractility, associated with a decreased ability to relax a muscle after contraction. May be congenital or acquired as a consequence of injury or disease. Percussion of a myotonic muscle produces a strong contraction that will be visible as an elevation beneath the skin.
Nystagmus	Involuntary, rapid, back-and-forth movements of the eye. May be horizontal, vertical, or rotatory in direction and be continuous or intermittent. May be provoked by changes in head position or direction of gaze. Many different kinds of nystagmus have been described. Frequently seen in association with disease involving the vestibular apparatus but may also be seen with diseases involving central nervous system structures including the cerebellum.
Opisthotonus	A strong and sustained contraction of the extensor muscles of the neck and trunk, producing a rigid, hyperextended posture. May also involve the extensor muscles of the shoulder, hip girdle, and proximal limbs.
Rigidity	Excessive muscle activity involving agonist and antagonist muscle groups together in such a way that stiffness and inflexibility results. Passive stretching of a rigid muscle is accompanied by a sudden, brief relaxation followed by a resumption of contraction, giving the examiner a sense of a "cogwheel" type of movement. Rigidity of the cogwheel type is frequently seen in patients with Parkinson's disease.
Tics	Involuntary, compulsive, repetitive, stereotyped movements, which generally appear purposeful and usually involve the face or shoulders. Patients may be able to suppress the irresistible urge to move for a while, but sooner or later the urge becomes too great and movement occurs, always intruding into the ongoing, otherwise normal behavior. Movements are most commonly seen in the face, where they frequently appear as blinking, lip smacking, grinning, licking, or wrinkling of the nose or forehead. Spontaneous vocalizations may also be heard. Tics are a frequent manifestation of the syndrome of Gilles de la Tourette.
Titubation	A shaking of the trunk or more commonly of the head, making it appear to be unsteady on the neck. May also involve the limbs, producing instability or a staggering gait. Seen in some patients with lesions involving the cerebellum.
Torticollis	A sustained state of contraction of the neck muscles producing rotation or tilting of the head.
Tremor	Involuntary, rhythmic contractions of muscles, producing the appearance of trembling or quivering. May be present at rest, with movement, or with efforts to sustain a fixed position. Numerous types of tremor have been described, of which some of the more common are rest tremor, essential tremor, postural or sustention tremor, and action or intention tremor.

(Continued)

TABLE 9 *Descriptive Characteristics of Selected Motor Disturbances (Continued)*

Trismus	A sustained contraction of the muscles of mastication, making it difficult or impossible for the patient to open the mouth. Often seen in association with diseases involving the motor division of the trigeminal nerve.

spindles are associated with increased muscle tone, and hyposensitive muscle spindles are associated with decreased muscle tone.

Muscle tone can be evaluated in several ways. The easiest is for the examiner to move the patient's limbs through their normal range of motion while the patient attempts to remain completely relaxed. Some patients may need to be encouraged to relax completely and allow the examiner to do all the work. Muscle tone will be difficult to evaluate by this method if the patient is unable for one reason or another to cooperate fully. All four limbs should be tested so that the two sides and the upper and lower limbs on each side can be compared. The examiner's task is to assess the freedom of movement at each joint. Attention should be focused on the relative amount of resistance to passive movement. Note that the evaluation of muscle tone is based on the examiner's *perception* of the presence or absence of resistance to *passive* movement.

The first judgment to be made is whether the relative resistance to passive movement is the same on both sides (symmetric) or different (asymmetric). Making this judgment may take a little practice but should not be difficult. A clinical finding of symmetric muscle tone does not necessarily rule out neurologic disease, but clearly asymmetric tone always indicates some degree of neurologic dysfunction. If muscle tone is judged to be asymmetric, it will be necessary to determine which is the abnormal side. That is to say, is the side that offers less resistance normal, suggesting that the contralateral side is hypertonic, or is the side with greater resistance normal, suggesting that the other side is hypotonic? Clinical experience and careful attention to the results of other tests of motor function will provide the answer.

In some cases, muscle tone may be laterally symmetric but increased or decreased in either the upper or lower limbs. Differences in muscle tone between the upper and lower limbs generally suggest injury or disease involving the spinal cord at or below the level of the cervical enlargement. Complete lesions are usually characterized by symmetric alterations in muscle tone, whereas incomplete lesions may result in asymmetric changes in tone.

Clinical examination may reveal muscle tone to be normal, decreased, or increased. As indicated earlier, normal muscle tone is the degree or strength of contraction that characterizes normally innervated, resting skeletal muscle and is the result of the ongoing activation of a certain number of motor units. It is difficult to describe the clinical experience of normal muscle tone other than to point out that there is no detectable resistance to passive movement. The "clinical feel" of normal muscle tone is best appreciated when compared with the more easily defined conditions of decreased and increased tone.

Muscle tone is decreased when excitatory influences on alpha motor neurons are reduced or lost. Excitatory input to alpha motor neurons is derived from both segmental and suprasegmental sources. Segmental sources include local interneurons and dorsal root ganglion cells that transmit impulses from muscle spindles and sensory receptors in the skin and visceral structures. Suprasegmental sources of excitatory input include certain brainstem nuclei and cortical regions described earlier as being the source of upper motor neurons.

By far the most powerful excitatory influence on motor unit activity is the Ia fiber transmitting impulses from muscle spindles located in the motor unit itself. When this powerful influence is lost through injury or disease, excitation of the motor unit produced by muscle stretch is also lost. The result is a greatly reduced level of firing of the affected lower motor neurons with a concomitant reduction in the activity of the motor unit. The clinical expression of this condition is either reduced muscle tone (hypotonia) or absent muscle tone (atonia). Because lower motor neurons are not being activated in sufficient numbers to maintain normal muscle tone, patients with reduced or absent muscle tone may also be weak. In addition, as we will discuss later, muscle stretch reflexes in these patients will be reduced (hyporeflexia) or lost (areflexia).

Muscle tone can also be decreased as a consequence of the loss of certain upper motor neuron influences on the motor unit. Frequently, patients with lesions involving the cerebellum may demonstrate a degree of reduced muscle tone. This reduction is usually on the side ipsilateral to the side of cerebellar disease.

Muscle tone is increased when motor units are overly active, either because inhibitory influences on lower motor neurons are reduced or lost or because excitatory influences are relatively increased in their effect. Because segmental afferent influences on lower motor neurons are functionally excitatory, muscle tone is not increased in patients with lesions involving peripheral nervous system structures. Clinically, increased muscle tone occurs only in response to lesions involving central nervous system structures. Destructive lesions produce increased muscle tone (hypertonia) by effectively eliminating or reducing inhibitory influences on lower motor neurons. Therefore, when a muscle or group of muscles in a patient with hypertonia is passively stretched, the excitatory effect mediated by muscle spindle stretch receptors is not modulated or counterbalanced by the absent inhibitory influences, and the result is a clinically detectable resistance to passive movement that is not present in the normal individual. Irritative lesions can also cause increased muscle tone if the irritated neurons normally exert an excitatory effect on lower motor neurons.

Increased muscle tone has different characteristics depending on the nature and location of the lesion producing it. In the case of lesions involving the internal capsule, for example, the resistance to passive stretch depends on the speed and direction of passive movement. That is, the faster a muscle is stretched, the greater the resistance to stretch it will produce. Such resistance to passive movement is referred to as *spasticity*, and is characterized by increasing resistance up to a point, after which there is a sudden relaxation or giving way. The phenomenon is commonly called the "clasp-knife response," and the term "clasp-knife spasticity" is frequently used. Patients with spasticity usually also demonstrate weakness and hyperactive muscle stretch reflexes. In patients who have suffered a stroke, the resistance offered by the shoulder adductors and internal rotators, elbow flexors, forearm pronators, and wrist and finger flexors is typically greater than that offered by their antagonist muscles. In the lower limb, a greater resistance to passive movement is usually seen in the hip extensors and adductors, knee extensors, and ankle and foot plantar flexors, muscle groups that are used for standing and walking.

Another type of increased muscle tone is seen in patients with diseases involving certain of the basal nuclei. In Parkinson's disease, for example, the increased muscle tone is characterized by slight giving way followed almost immediately by a return to the former motor unit hyperactivity. The serial increase-decrease-increase-decrease in resistance to passive movement that occurs throughout the range of motion is likened to pulling a lever over a cogwheel, and the phenomenon is therefore commonly referred to as *cogwheel rigidity*. Rigidity of this type differs from spasticity in that it generally involves all muscles or muscle groups in a particular limb equally.

Not all resistance to passive movement is the result of increased muscle tone, however. Muscle contractures, diseases of joints (arthropathies), and pain can all produce limitations in or resistance to passive movement. Contractures can be palpated and become more apparent as the muscle is progressively stretched. The resistance to stretch associated with contractures increases with continued efforts to further lengthen the muscle. Such effects also may provoke a significant amount of pain. At no point will the resistance to stretch lessen or give way unless there is disruption or physical damage to the anatomic structures responsible for the contracture.

Joint diseases can also limit or impair passive range of motion. Patients with inflammatory joint disease generally limit their joint movements voluntarily and resist attempts by the examiner to move their inflamed or painful joints through their full ranges of motion. The bony fusion of a joint will obviously produce a resistance to passive movement, but ankylosis of a joint is not likely to be confused with increased muscle tone.

Muscle tone can also be assessed by palpation of the muscle belly. This technique may be particularly useful in assessing muscle tone in the lower limbs, which may be difficult to move passively through a range of motion. Hypotonic or atonic muscles will feel softer and compress more easily when squeezed. This should be expected because hypotonia is the result of reduced activity of motor units. In contrast, hypertonic muscles will feel as though they are in a state of contraction. Even when the patient is relaxed as much as possible, muscles will seem harder than normal. The ability to evaluate muscle tone by means of palpation will require some skill and practice. Experience can be easily gained if the examiner takes the time to palpate muscles while evaluating tone by moving the limbs through their range of motion. Comparisons and correlations can easily be made by this simple technique. There is no substitute for hands-on practice in evaluating muscle tone.

Muscle Strength

Muscle strength is a measure of the force that a muscle can produce, either to move a body part about a joint or to resist movement about a joint. Strength is related to the number of motor units recruited for a particular task, which in turn is related to the number of alpha motor neurons activated by segmental or suprasegmental sources. Strength can be reduced as a consequence of both neurologic and non-neurologic disease processes. Neurologic causes of weakness include lesions involving the central nervous system structures or components of the peripheral nervous system. Common non-neurologic causes of reduced strength include primary diseases of muscle and conditions that affect neuromuscular transmission. Pain is a frequently overlooked but not uncommon cause of weakness.

Strength testing involves having the patient make a maximal voluntary effort to contract a muscle or muscle group while the examiner makes a judgment regarding the force of contraction. The ability to assess muscle strength accurately requires a working knowledge of the origin, insertion, action, and innervation of the muscles being tested.

In addition, a grading system is needed to differentiate among various degrees of strength of contraction. A six-category grading system is commonly used to evaluate muscle strength. Different terms have been used to refer to different strength grades, but these are easily equated. A listing of the most common methods of grading muscle strength is presented in Table 10, which describes the criteria that define each grade.

Strength testing is helpful in evaluating suspected peripheral mononeuropathies, polyneuropathies, plexopathies, and radiculopathies. Careful testing can provide precise information about the exact location and extent of nerve damage. In patients with suspected lesions or injuries involving the central nervous system, muscle testing can be helpful in determining the location or site of the lesion. Muscle testing in patients with suspected lesions in the brain, brainstem, or spinal cord can give an indication of the level and side of the lesion. A brief description of techniques for evaluating the strength of functionally organized groups of muscles is provided here. Techniques used to evaluate the strength of muscles of the head and neck have already been described in connection with the evaluation of cranial nerve function (see Chapter 4) and are not reviewed here. This discussion focuses on simple techniques that can be used to measure the strength of muscles and muscle groups innervated by spinal nerves. Test procedures are described in terms of the movements that should be evaluated. The major muscles involved in each movement are listed, along with the peripheral nerves and nerve roots that convey motor fibers to those muscles.

Upper Limb

Shoulder elevation (shoulder shrug).
 Upper trapezius (spinal accessory nerve, cranial nerve XI)
 Levator scapulae (C_3–C_4, dorsal scapular nerve, C_5)
 Patient, sitting with arms at sides, raises shoulders toward ears.
  Examiner attempts to depress shoulders by pushing down from
  above.
Shoulder abduction.
 Deltoid (axillary nerve, C_5–C_6)
 Supraspinatus (suprascapular nerve, C_5–C_6)
 Patient, sitting with arm at side and elbow flexed to 90 degrees,
  abducts arm through full range of motion. Examiner attempts to
  adduct arm from 90 degrees of abduction.
Shoulder retraction (scapular adduction).
 Rhomboid major and minor (dorsal scapular nerve, C_5)
 Patient, sitting with arms at sides, pulls shoulders back (retracts
  shoulders). Examiner, standing behind the patient, attempts to
  push shoulder forward while palpating rhomboid muscles.

TABLE 10 *Methods of Grading Muscle Strength*

Word	Number	Percent	Performance Criteria
Normal	5	100	Full range of motion against gravity with maximum resistance
Good	4	75	Full range of motion against gravity with some resistance
Fair	3	50	Full range of motion against gravity only
Poor	2	25	Full range of motion with gravity eliminated
Trace	1	10	Palpable or visual evidence of slight contraction without joint movement
Zero	0	0	No palpable or visual evidence of muscle contraction

Shoulder protraction (scapular abduction).
   Serratus anterior (long thoracic nerve, C_5-C_7)
   Patient, sitting, reaches forward with both arms, elbows extended.
      Examiner attempts to push extended arm backward while looking
      for winging of the scapula.
Shoulder flexion.
   Anterior deltoid (axillary nerve, C_5-C_6)
   Coracobrachialis (musculocutaneous nerve, C_6-C_7)
   Patient, sitting with arm at side, elbow fully flexed, and forearm
      supinated, flexes arm through full range of motion. Examiner
      attempts to push arm into extension, back to starting position.
Shoulder extension.
   Latissimus dorsi (thoracodorsal nerve, C_6-C_8)
   Teres major (lower subscapular nerve, C_5-C_7)
   Patient, lying prone with arm at side, elbow extended, and forearm
      pronated, extends arm (lifts arm off table or bed). Examiner
      attempts to push arm into flexion, back to starting position.
Shoulder external rotation.
   Infraspinatus (suprascapular nerve, C_5-C_6)
   Teres minor (axillary nerve, C_5-C_6)
   Patient lying prone, with shoulder abducted to 90 degrees and
      forearm hanging vertically off side of table, rotates shoulder to
      raise forearm forward to the horizontal position. Examiner
      attempts to push forearm down to vertical starting position.
Shoulder internal rotation.
   Subscapularis (upper and lower subscapular nerves, C_5-C_7)
   Latissimus dorsi (thoracodorsal nerve, C_6-C_8)
   Pectoralis major (medial and lateral pectoral nerves, C_5-T_1)
   Teres major (lower subscapular nerve, C_5-C_7)
   Patient lying prone with shoulder abducted to 90 degrees and
      forearm hanging vertically off side of table, rotates shoulder to

raise forearm backward to horizontal position. Examiner attempts to push forearm down to vertical starting position.

Elbow flexion.

Biceps brachii (musculocutaneous nerve, C_5–C_6)

Brachialis (musculocutaneous nerve, C_5–C_6)

Patient, sitting with arm at side, elbow fully extended, and forearm supinated, flexes elbow through full range of motion. Examiner attempts to pull elbow into extension.

Elbow extension.

Triceps brachii (radial nerve, C_6–C_8)

Patient, lying supine with shoulder flexed to 90 degrees and elbow flexed, extends elbow through full range of motion. Examiner attempts to push elbow into flexion.

Forearm supination.

Supinator (radial nerve, C_5–C_6)

Biceps brachii (musculocutaneous nerve, C_5–C_6)

Patient, sitting with arm at side, elbow flexed to 90 degrees, and forearm fully pronated, supinates forearm (turns palm up). Examiner attempts to turn forearm into pronation (palm-down position).

Forearm pronation.

Pronator teres (median nerve, C_6–C_7)

Pronator quadratus (median nerve, C_8–T_1)

Patient, sitting with arm at side, elbow flexed to 90 degrees, and forearm fully supinated, pronates forearm (turns palm down). Examiner attempts to turn forearm into supination (palm-up position).

Wrist extension.

Extensor carpi radialis longus (radial nerve, C_6–C_7)

Extensor carpi radialis brevis (radial nerve, C_6–C_7)

Extensor carpi ulnaris (radial nerve, C_7–C_8)

Patient, sitting with arm at side, elbow flexed to 90 degrees, forearm in midposition, and wrist fully flexed, extends wrist through full range of motion. Examiner attempts to push extended wrist into flexion.

Wrist flexion.

Flexor carpi radialis (median nerve, C_6–C_7)

Flexor carpi ulnaris (median nerve, C_8–T_1)

Patient, sitting with arm at side, elbow flexed to 90 degrees, forearm in midposition, and wrist fully extended, flexes wrist through full range of motion. Examiner attempts to push wrist into extension.

Finger extension.

Extensor digitorum (radial nerve, C_6–C_8)

Extensor digiti minimi (radial nerve, C_6-C_8)
Extensor indicis proprius (radial nerve, C_6-C_8)
Patient, sitting with arm at side, elbow flexed to 90 degrees, forearm in midposition, and fingers fully flexed, extends fingers through full range of motion. Examiner attempts to push fingers into flexion.

Finger flexion.
Flexor digitorum profundus (median nerve, C_7-T_1, ulnar nerve, C_7-T_1)
Flexor digitorum superficialis (median nerve, C_7-T_1)
Lumbricales (median nerve, C_7-T_1, ulnar nerve, C_7-T_1)
Patient, sitting with arm at side, elbow flexed to 90 degrees, forearm in midposition, and fingers fully extended, flexes fingers through full range of motion. Examiner attempts to pull fingers into extension.

Finger abduction.
Dorsal interossei (ulnar nerve, C_8-T_1)
Patient, sitting with arm at side, elbow flexed to 90 degrees, and forearm and wrist in comfortable position with fingers extended but together, spreads fingers apart. Examiner attempts to push adjacent fingers together.

Finger adduction.
Palmar interossei (ulnar nerve, C_8-T_1)
Patient, sitting with arm at side, elbow flexed to 90 degrees, and forearm and wrist in comfortable position with fingers extended and spread, brings fingers together. Examiner attempts to spread extended fingers apart.

A useful screening test for distal upper limb strength is for the examiner to ask the patient to squeeze hard on two of the examiner's fingers, placed in the patient's palm. This test is useful also in assessing whether the patient is able to release grasp quickly and on command. Inability to do so may indicate myotonia.

Weakness of the muscles of the upper limb is commonly seen in patients who have suffered a stroke and may be associated with the sign of pronator drift. To detect pronator drift, the patient is asked to close the eyes and extend the arms forward in a parallel fashion with the palms up. The patient should attempt to maintain this position for 15 to 30 seconds. Pronator drift is present when the supinated forearm gradually rotates toward the midposition. Not infrequently, the weak upper limb will also begin to fall from the forward extended position. Weakness and pronator drift seen in association with stroke are evident on the side contralateral to the vascular accident.

Lower Limb

Hip flexion.

Psoas major (L_2, L_3)
Iliacus (L_2, L_3)
Patient, sitting upright with hips and knees flexed to 90 degrees, lifts thigh, bringing knee up as far as possible. Examiner attempts to push thigh back down to starting position.

Hip extension.

Gluteus maximus (inferior gluteal nerve, L_5, S_1–S_2)
Patient, lying prone with knee flexed to 90 degrees, lifts thigh from surface of table or bed. Examiner attempts to push thigh back to starting position.

Hip abduction.

Gluteus medius (superior gluteal nerve, L_4–L_5, S_1)
Gluteus minimus (superior gluteal nerve, L_4–L_5, S_1)
Patient, lying on side with uppermost hip and knee in full extension, lifts thigh and leg toward ceiling, maintaining hip and knee in extension. Examiner attempts to push limb back to starting position.

Hip adduction.

Adductor magnus (obturator nerve, L_2–L_4)
Adductor brevis (obturator nerve, L_2–L_4)
Adductor longus (obturator nerve, L_2–L_4)
Patient is lying on side with both hips and knees fully extended. Examiner lifts uppermost lower limb, thereby abducting the thighs. Patient is asked to raise lower thigh off the surface of the bed or table to bring it in contact with the upper thigh, raised attempts to push lowermost thigh back to starting position.

Knee extension.

Quadriceps femoris (femoral nerve, L_2–L_4)
Patient, sitting upright with hips and knees flexed to 90 degrees, straightens leg to bring knee into full extension. Examiner attempts to push leg back to starting position.

Knee flexion.

Biceps femoris (sciatic nerve, L_5–S_2)
Semitendinosus (sciatic nerve, L_4–S_2)
Semimembranous (sciatic nerve, L_4–S_2)
Patient, lying prone with hips and knees fully extended, bends knee through full range of motion. Examiner attempts to pull leg back to starting position.

Ankle dorsiflexion.

Anterior tibialis (deep peroneal nerve, L_4–S_1)
Extensor hallucis longus (deep peroneal nerve, L_4–S_1)

Extensor digitorum longus (deep peroneal nerve, L_4-S_1)
Patient, sitting or lying supine with knee extended and ankle resting comfortably, dorsiflexes foot through full range of motion. Examiner attempts to push foot into plantar flexion.
Ankle plantar flexion.
Gastrocnemius (tibial nerve, S_1-S_2)
Posterior tibialis (tibial nerve, L_5-S_1)
Soleus (tibial nerve, S_1-S_2)
Patient, sitting or lying supine with knee extended and ankle resting comfortably, plantar-flexes foot through full range of motion. Examiner attempts to push foot into dorsiflexion.

The tests for muscle strength just described are relatively simple and easy to perform. The descriptions provided are those that would yield grades of normal (5), good (4), and fair (3). A grade of poor (2) requires that movement be tested in the gravity-eliminated position, which would require some readjustment of the patient's position. If accuracy to that degree is required, the clinician will need to become familiar with some of the more subtle and specific aspects of manual muscle testing. Physical and occupational therapists are well trained to perform and interpret the results of these more complicated test procedures.

Strength testing is important in the evaluation of suspected lesions involving muscle or peripheral nerve, plexus, or spinal nerve roots. Indeed, these tests were originally developed for use in evaluating patients with diseases involving lower motor neurons and the motor unit. Their usefulness in evaluating patients with suspected upper motor neuron disease may be somewhat limited because such lesions may also affect muscle tone. They can be used, however, for the more general purpose of assessing changes that might occur over time after central nervous system injury or in response to focused therapeutic intervention.

The question invariably arises as to how many individual muscles or muscle groups should be tested in the neurologic examination. The answer depends entirely on the clinical situation and the specific needs of the examiner. Sometimes a very detailed evaluation may be required, such as in a patient with a suspected peripheral neuropathy, polyneuropathy, or radiculopathy. At other times a more limited assessment may be adequate, such as in a patient suspected of having suffered a stroke. In my experience, however, having more information about a particular patient seems better than having too little. We have all had the experience of failing to obtain information during an initial examination that later proves essential. Plenty of experience is needed for an examiner to make decisions about how much and what type of information will permit an accurate assessment of a patient's condition.

The test procedures just described are best learned early in the clinician's career. They are sufficient in number and specificity to permit the examiner to identify subtle degrees of weakness and to distinguish whether the weakness is caused by disease involving peripheral nerves, nerve plexuses, or nerve roots.

The degree and distribution of weakness have important implications regarding the precise location of a suspected lesion. Differences in strength between the two sides is an important clinical observation. Weakness associated with decreased tone is a typical feature of lower motor neuron or peripheral nerve disease. A lesser degree of weakness associated with increased muscle tone is commonly seen in patients with central nervous system or upper motor neuron diseases.

Coordination

The cerebellum plays an important role in motor behavior and the word *coordination* is frequently used in connection with cerebellar function. Clinical evidence suggests that a major function of the cerebellum is to orchestrate muscle activity so that movements that collectively make up normal behavior are carried out smoothly and sequentially. Generally speaking, disorders of coordination are not seen at rest but occur when the individual engages in some type of volitional activity.

A number of tests can be used to evaluate cerebellar function. The *finger-to-nose test* is used to evaluate cerebellar control of upper limb muscles. The patient is asked to alternately touch his or her nose and the tip of the examiner's finger, which is held steady at some distance in front of the patient. It is important that the examiner's finger be held far enough in front of the patient so that the patient must fully extend the arm to reach it. The examiner carefully observes the patient's hand as it is moved back and forth between the two endpoints. Neurologically intact individuals should be able to perform these movements smoothly, being able to touch both targets without difficulty. The movements should be direct and precise. Patients with cerebellar disease will have difficulty performing this task. The arm and hand movements will appear unsteady or shaky, giving the impression that the patient is attempting to correct or compensate for a misdirected movement. The inability to perform the task properly is referred to as *dysmetria*. The movement itself is often characterized as ataxic. The tremor-like movements may be seen during the entire time when the limb is in motion or, in some patients, only as the finger approaches the target. These types of movement disorders are referred to as *action* or *intention tremors*. Action tremors are seen in patients with lesions involving the ipsilateral cerebellar hemisphere.

The *rebound phenomenon* may also be seen in patients with cerebellar disease. This sign is elicited by having the patient reach with both arms toward the ceiling and then very quickly bring both arms down to the horizontal position. The normal individual should be able to bring the arms to a sudden stop in the forward position without demonstrating any bounce or rebound-type movement. The patient with cerebellar disease may have difficulty in initiating a rapid, downward movement of the arms from the overhead position and may be unable to suddenly stop the downward movement. The attempt to stop the downward movement abruptly is immediately followed by a brief rebound-type movement in the opposite direction.

Another test of cerebellar function is to assess skill in performing rapidly alternating movements. This can be done by asking the patient to rapidly pat his or her thigh alternately with the palm and the back of the hand. The task requires that the patient rapidly supinate and pronate the forearm. Normal individuals should be able to perform these movements rapidly and rhythmically. The movements of patients with cerebellar disease will be slow and dysrhythmic.

An alternative form of this test is to ask the patient to rapidly tap the tip of the thumb with the tip of the index finger. Again, patients with cerebellar disease will have difficulty in performing these movements. The inability to perform rapidly alternating movements or other simple motor tasks involving the rapid contraction and relaxation of agonist and antagonist muscles is referred to as *dysdiadochokinesia*.

Cerebellar influence on lower limb motor function can be evaluated by asking the patient to place his or her heel on the knee and to then slide it distally toward the foot along the anterior border of the tibia. In the normal individual, the heel should move in a smooth, straight course toward the foot, without sliding off the tibial crest. In patients with cerebellar disease, the descent of the heel will be unsteady, and contact between the heel and the leg will not be maintained. The inability to perform this maneuver properly indicates *dysmetria*.

Another technique to evaluate the lower limb coordination of patients with suspected cerebellar disease who are in bed or lying down is to instruct them to raise one foot and trace a figure-8 pattern in the air. This task requires coordination of hip girdle and proximal limb muscles. Normal individuals are able to perform this maneuver with little difficulty. The movements seen in patients with cerebellar dysfunction are slow and ataxic. The task will be done poorly and with great effort and difficulty.

The ability to perform rapid alternating movements involving the lower limb can be evaluated by asking the patient to rapidly tap his or her foot on the floor. Slow movements with uneven rhythm are indicative of dysdiadochokinesia and are not uncommon in patients with lesions involving the cerebellum.

As suggested previously, the ability to coordinate muscle activity so that movements are appropriate in terms of their amplitude, direction, and velocity requires the participation of the cerebellum. The tests of cerebellar function just described focus on coordination of the limbs, although movements produced by axial muscles also can be ataxic and uncoordinated. Clinical and experimental evidence indicates that the lateral or hemispheric portion of the cerebellum is most involved with coordination of limb muscle groups. Therefore, lesions involving the cerebellar hemispheres are likely to be associated with incoordination of limb movements. In addition, because of the anatomic connections of the cerebellum, signs of cerebellar hemisphere dysfunction such as dysmetria, dysdiadochokinesia, and intention tremor will be seen on the ipsilateral side. Lesions involving the vermal portions of the cerebellum are more likely to affect trunk muscle groups, leaving limb coordination relatively intact.

Station and Gait

The final component of the motor systems examination is an evaluation of station and gait. Station can be thought of as a measure of postural control. In a practical sense, *station* refers to the ability to stand upright without moving, using muscle activity only to overcome the force of gravity. *Gait* refers to the processes of recruiting and coordinating the activity of various muscle groups of lower limbs, upper limbs, and trunk to produce the act of walking. Stated differently, gait refers to the ability to perturb posture in an intentional and purposeful way to move from one place to another.

Station is evaluated simply by observing the patient while he or she stands. The patient should be asked to stand with the feet together, the arms hanging comfortably at the sides, and the head facing forward with the eyes open. Normal individuals should be able to maintain this position without moving or swaying about. Patients who sway from side to side or front to back or who lean or fall to one side *with the eyes open* may have disease involving the cerebellum. If the patient consistently falls to one side while attempting to stand upright, cerebellar disease may be suspected on the ipsilateral side, although unilateral muscle weakness may also cause a patient to fall to one side. If the clinician is uncertain as to the cause of the patient's falling, further tests of strength and cerebellar function would be indicated.

The Romberg test is performed by having the patient stand upright with the feet together and the head facing forward with the eyes open as described above. The patient is then asked *to close the eyes* and to maintain the upright standing position. Normal individuals should be able to continue standing with the eyes closed without swaying or falling. The Romberg test in this situation would be reported as negative. If the patient is able to stand motionless with the eyes open, but loses his or her balance or begins to fall *with the eyes closed*, the test is said to be positive. A positive Romberg test suggests disease involving the dorsal columns of the spinal cord. So long as the patient can use visual cues to control the muscle activity necessary for standing, he or she is able to stand without wavering, but if visual cues are eliminated, the patient is forced to rely heavily on proprioceptive information transmitted to the brain by way of the dorsal columns. Therefore, patients have difficulty in standing if conduction in the dorsal columns is impaired.

Gait is evaluated by watching the patient walk. Patients should be asked to walk some distance at a comfortable pace in their natural manner. The clinician should observe components of gait such as speed, step length, foot placement, center of gravity relative to foot placement, arm swing, and associated trunk movements. Although characteristics of gait vary somewhat from individual to individual, it is generally not difficult to recognize an abnormal gait pattern. It may require some experience, however, to determine the nature and probable cause of a particular abnormal gait pattern.

Certain disease processes are characterized by fairly specific gait abnormalities. Examples of common gait abnormalities include the circumducted or hemiplegic gait seen in patients following cerebrovascular accidents, the festinating gait seen in patients with Parkinson's disease, the steppage gait seen in patients with disease of the dorsal columns of the spinal cord, the ataxic gait associated with lesions of the cerebellum, and the antalgic gait seen in patients who have an altered gait pattern because of pain. The ability to identify these gait disturbances correctly comes only from the careful observation of many patients with various conditions that produce gait disturbances.

Tandem walking is a useful way of bringing out certain problems related to equilibrium and coordination. Patients are asked to walk a short distance by placing one foot directly in front of the other, heel to toe, as if walking on a thin line. Normal individuals have little difficulty in walking this way. Patients with cerebellar disease tend to lose their balance as they attempt to walk tandem fashion and may employ all sorts of arm and trunk movements to avoid falling. Gait may also be affected by weakness or pain, both of which produce patterns of walking that are easily distinguished.

If the evaluation of gait seems difficult at first, it is generally not because the examiner lacks an understanding of the neural bases of motor function, but rather because not enough careful attention has been paid to the many components of walking as they appear in the normal population. The reader is encouraged to study people when they walk, paying close attention to the various movements of all body parts from head to foot.

SUMMARY

Abnormalities of motor function are generally recognized by the patient and fairly easy for the observant clinician to identify and characterize. Some motor abnormalities are little more than a nuisance, whereas others may cause major disability. Disease involving the motor systems may occur in isolation or may be accompanied by disease or dysfunction involving other neurologic or non-neurologic systems. As with other parts of the neurologic evaluation, skill and competence in evaluating motor function will be acquired only as a result of thoughtful and reflective practice.

6

REFLEXES

A reflex is a relatively invariant response to a particular stimulus. Many physiologic functions involved in the maintenance of homeostasis are regulated by reflex mechanisms. In addition, a large number of somatic and visceral motor behaviors that help ensure survival of the individual occur reflexly. One might view the retention and refinement of reflex mechanisms throughout evolution as a means of relieving the individual of the need to be constantly attentive to a continually changing environment.

We frequently think of reflexes as simple motor behaviors over which we have little or no control. In reality, reflexes and reflex behaviors can be quite complex and can be influenced by a variety of metabolic, physiologic, or pathologic processes. We can use these characteristics of reflex behavior to our advantage when examining patients. For example, a number of reflexes are mediated only by brainstem or spinal cord structures. These reflexes may be particularly helpful in evaluating the unconscious patient. In addition, the predictable changes in some reflex responses as a result of injury or disease can provide the examiner with useful information about the location or nature of the reflex-altering process.

FUNCTIONAL ANATOMY

The reflex arc consists of four essential elements: a receptor or transducer, the afferent limb, the efferent limb, and the effector. The *receptor* is that part of the reflex mechanism that converts the energy of the stimulus into nerve impulses. Any of the receptors commonly discussed in courses in general neuroanatomy or neurophysiology can be part of a reflex mechanism. The *afferent limb* is the neuron that conveys nerve impulses from the receptor to the central nervous system. The cell bodies of these neurons are part of the peripheral nervous system and compose dorsal root ganglia and sensory cranial nerve ganglia. These neurons are either pseudounipolar or bipolar in structure, with a peripheral process that extends toward and makes contact with the receptor and a central process that enters the central nervous system. The central processes of neurons serving as the afferent limb of spinal reflexes form the dorsal root. The *efferent limb* is represented by the cell body and axon of a motor neuron. Reflex responses involving the contraction of skeletal muscles use alpha motor neurons and their axons as the efferent limb, whereas reflexes characterized by the activity of smooth muscle, cardiac muscle, and glands use autonomic preganglionic and postganglionic neurons as the efferent limb. The *effector* is the structure innervated by the efferent limb, the action of which constitutes the reflex response. As indicated above, the reflex response can be the contraction of skeletal, smooth, or cardiac muscle or the secretion of a glandular product.

In addition to these four essential elements of the reflex arc, interneurons interposed between the afferent and efferent limb play an important part in many reflex responses. Indeed, it is the excitatory and inhibitory effects on lower motor neurons mediated by interneurons that are largely responsible for the range of responses that characterize normal and abnormal reflex behavior.

Reflex testing provides an opportunity to evaluate the functional integrity of relatively small segments of the nervous system. For this reason, the results have potential value in terms of both diagnosis and localization of disease. The most useful reflex tests are those that involve the fewest components. These simple reflexes are generally easy to elicit and are not easily controlled or influenced by the patient. In addition, it is easier to interpret an abnormal finding because only a limited number of neurons and other structures are involved.

Reflexes are classified in a number of ways. This chapter considers two types of reflexes that are essential components of the neurologic examination: muscle stretch reflexes and cutaneous reflexes, each named according to the stimulus used to elicit them. Abnormal reflex responses that suggest injury or disease will be considered within the appropriate category. Reflexes involving the cranial nerves were considered in Chapter 4 and will not be reviewed here except for a few pathologic reflexes that are typically evaluated during this phase of the neurologic examination.

MUSCLE STRETCH REFLEXES

Muscle stretch reflexes form the basis of normal motor behavior. They are characterized by contraction of a skeletal muscle in response to a stimulus that causes lengthening of that muscle. Stretch reflexes are an integral part of mechanisms used to control posture and regulate movement. They help ensure that the length of a muscle is kept constant in the face of a changing load. In the weight-bearing limbs, stretch reflexes mediate muscle contraction necessary to overcome the force of gravity acting on joints while standing and walking. Moreover, they operate largely at a segmental level, thereby leaving higher levels of the nervous system free to engage in other activities.

Functional Anatomy

The components of the muscle stretch reflex (Fig. 22) are the *muscle spindle*, which is sensitive to changes in length of a muscle; the type Ia and II *afferent nerve fibers*, which transmit impulses from the muscle spindle to the central nervous system; the *alpha motor neuron*, which innervates the skeletal muscle in which the muscle spindle is located; and the *skeletal muscle* itself. The adequate stimulus for the muscle stretch reflex is lengthening of the skeletal muscle. The response includes excitation of alpha motor neurons that innervate the stretched muscle, together with inhibition of alpha motor neurons that innervate antagonistic muscles.

A key element of the muscle stretch reflex is the muscle spindle. As described earlier, muscle spindles are specialized receptor structures composed of intrafusal muscle cells. Muscle spindles are composed of 2 to 12 intrafusal muscle cells encapsulated in a connective tissue sheath, the ends of which are attached to the perimysium of a skeletal muscle fascicle. This anatomic arrangement places the muscle spindle in parallel with the skeletal muscle with which it is associated. Because of this arrangement, the muscle spindle is affected by, and can respond to, both the relative static length of the skeletal muscle to which it is attached and

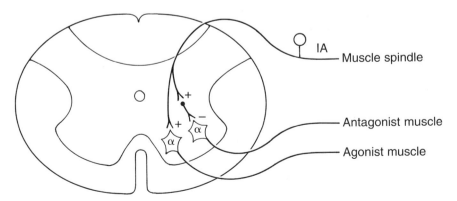

FIGURE 22. The afferent and efferent limbs of the muscle stretch (myotatic) reflex.

the rate at which the length of the muscle changes during contraction or lengthening.

Each intrafusal muscle cell has a central, equatorial region that is sensitive to elongation and two polar regions that contain the contractile proteins actin and myosin. The central, equatorial region contains the peripheral endings of the type Ia and type II afferent fibers. These endings are sensitive to changes in length of the muscle spindle. The polar, contractile regions of the intrafusal muscle cell receive motor innervation by way of gamma motor neurons. Contraction or relaxation of the muscle fibers in the polar regions of the muscle spindle induced by changes in gamma motor neuron activity alters the sensitivity of the spindle to passive movement or contraction-induced changes in extrafusal muscle length. Because the muscle spindle is attached in parallel with the skeletal muscle, lengthening of the skeletal muscle will cause the muscle spindle to be stretched, which in turn will result in an increase in the number of action potentials transmitted centrally along type Ia and type II afferent fibers. The effect produced by an increase in the transmission of impulses along these axons is excitation of alpha motor neurons that innervate the originally lengthened skeletal muscle. Activation of the alpha motor neurons causes the skeletal muscle to contract, thereby limiting or prohibiting further increases in muscle length. At the same time, activation of inhibitory interneurons by way of collateral branches of type Ia and type II fibers causes hyperpolarization of the alpha motor neurons that innervate antagonist muscles (see Fig. 22). This latter effect lessens the likelihood that the antagonist muscle will contract to further lengthen the already stretched skeletal muscle. The muscle spindle and reflex mechanisms described are important in the regulation of muscle tone and various neural processes involved in the control of posture and movement.

Clinical Examinations

Rationale and Technique

In the clinical setting, it is possible to exploit this normal, relatively simple, and largely automatic response to muscle stretch. To do so, it would be necessary to devise a way of stretching a skeletal muscle and its associated muscle spindles. The technique commonly used to induce muscle stretch is percussion of the muscle tendon. Such a stimulus produces a brief stretch that is transmitted through the skeletal muscle to the muscle spindles located therein. A percussion hammer with a soft but firm rubber head is usually used for this purpose.

When the tendon of an extrafusal (skeletal) muscle is properly percussed, muscle fibers attached to the tendon will be briefly and simultaneously stretched a very short distance. The slight increase in length of the skeletal muscle fibers is sufficient to cause the muscle spindles located in the muscle to be stretched, and this in turn causes action potentials to be transmitted to the central nervous system. Because the stimulus is sudden and brief, the result will be a synchronous volley of nerve impulses transmitted along a relatively homogeneous population of myelinated afferent fibers. Because conduction velocity is rapid and essentially the same for all type Ia fibers, the afferent impulses produced by the brief stretch will reach the central nervous system quickly and essentially at the same time. Moreover, because Ia fibers make excitatory, monosynaptic contact with alpha motor neurons, the result is excitation of alpha motor neurons, followed immediately by a brief, twitch-like contraction of the innervated skeletal muscle.

The most powerful influence on alpha motor neuron activity is the Ia afferent fiber. This idea is best understood by considering two principles of neural organization. First is the principle of convergence and divergence. Anatomic studies have shown that, within the central nervous system, the central processes of Ia muscle spindle afferent fibers divide into numerous collateral branches, which make direct contact with each of the alpha motor neurons that innervate the skeletal muscle in question. This anatomic arrangement is referred to as *divergence*. In addition, each alpha motor neuron that innervates a particular skeletal muscle receives direct synaptic input from all muscle spindles located in that skeletal muscle. This phenomenon is referred to as *convergence*.

The second principle is that of spatial and temporal summation. *Spatial summation* of nerve impulses is achieved by virtue of the numerous synaptic endings on a motor neuron that are derived from muscle spindle afferent fibers. *Temporal summation* of nerve impulses is achieved because conduction velocity among Ia afferent fibers is remarkably homogeneous, and the stimulus used to elicit impulse transmission is delivered simultaneously to all muscle spindles located within a given muscle. The concepts of convergence and divergence and spatial and temporal summation explain why a brief, virtually imperceptible change in the length of a muscle can cause contraction of the muscle, whereas a slower but more extensive increase in muscle length, such as that produced by passively moving a limb through a range of motion, does not. Thus, the simultaneous activation of a number of alpha motor neurons, each of which conducts nerve impulses at a similar velocity, will lead to the simultaneous contraction of the skeletal muscle fibers innervated. This contraction can be seen or palpated, and its characteristics can inform the examiner as to the integrity of the neurons and other anatomic structures involved in the reflex.

The proper technique for eliciting muscle stretch reflexes involves

more than simply percussing a muscle tendon. Three general requirements must be met to evaluate a muscle stretch reflex response properly:

1. The patient must remain completely relaxed while being tested.
   Many patients must be instructed to let their muscles go limp and
   to relax as completely as possible. Some patients have difficulty in
   achieving a satisfactory level of relaxation, and it may be necessary to distract them by having them talk about something unrelated to the test or having them focus their attention elsewhere.
2. There must be an optimal amount of resting tension in the muscle
   to be tested. Such tension is usually achieved by placing the muscle in a resting position midway between its shortest and longest
   lengths.
3. The stimulus applied to the tendon must be adequate in terms of
   its duration and strength. It should be brief in duration and strong
   enough to induce a slight lengthening of the muscle fibers attached to the tendon. The percussion hammer and the way it is
   used are important in this regard. The hammer should be properly
   balanced, and the weight of the head should be sufficient for the
   force of impact to produce the desired muscle stretch. If the force
   of impact is too great or too little, the elicited response will be influenced accordingly. Skill in the use of the percussion hammer
   must be acquired through practice.

Occasional patients appear to be areflexic even when tested in the
proper manner. With these patients, it is necessary to employ a reinforcement technique before concluding that a particular reflex is absent. A
useful technique for reinforcing lower limb reflexes is to ask the patient
to clench the fists. The examiner must percuss the tendon immediately
after the patient clenches the fists, because the reinforcement effect is
brief. An alternative method is the Jendrassik maneuver, in which the patient is asked to interlock the hands in front of the chest and pull apart
without letting go. Again, the lower limb tendon to be percussed should
be tapped immediately after the patient begins to try to pull the hands
apart. Muscle stretch reflexes in the upper limbs can be reinforced by the
examiner asking the patient to squeeze the knees together immediately
before percussing the tendon. If for any reason these techniques cannot
be used, asking the patient to clench the teeth may be helpful.

The normal response to percussion of a tendon is a brief, twitch-like
contraction of the muscle. The characteristics of the response that are
important to note are its speed, vigor, and duration. When large muscles
or muscle groups are being tested, the muscle contraction elicited may
be sufficient to produce movement of the joint over which the muscle
acts. Such visible movements present the examiner with little difficulty in
judging the quality and magnitude of the reflex. However, if the reflex re-

sponse is reduced for some reason or if joint movement is restricted, the contraction, even with reinforcement, may not be sufficient to produce visible movement. It is then necessary to assess the reflex response by means of palpation. Reflex responses can be felt in a number of ways. For muscle stretch reflexes like the pectoral and biceps brachii reflexes, the examiner should gently press the tendon with a finger and then percuss the finger. In this way, the examiner will be able to feel a slight increase in tension in the tendon that occurs when the muscle contracts. An alternative method is to use a finger or hand to place the muscle under a slight tension before percussion. This technique is particularly useful in evaluating the Achilles tendon reflex and the jaw reflex. Finally, for some muscle stretch reflexes, such as the patellar tendon reflex, one can simply palpate the muscle belly in an effort to feel the stretch-induced muscle contraction. The important point to remember is that it is absolutely necessary to use the most sensitive method possible to detect muscle contraction in response to percussion-induced muscle stretch. The examiner must therefore be knowledgeable about these various techniques and skilled in their use.

Grading the reflex response is an important and necessary part of reflex testing. The grading system must have enough categories to distinguish real and meaningful differences among responses, but not so many that it becomes difficult to choose among them. The six-point scale shown in Table 11 is quite adequate for documenting muscle stretch reflex responses.

Grades 4+ and 5+ represent clearly abnormal reflex responses in which the degree of contraction is excessive and clonus (see next paragraph) is present. These grades are further characterized by a decrease

TABLE 11 *Grading Scale for Muscle Stretch Reflexes*

Grade	Evaluation	Response Characteristics
0	Absent	No visible or palpable muscle contraction with reinforcement.
1+	Hyporeflexia	Slight or sluggish muscle contraction with little or no joint movement. Reinforcement may be required to elicit a reflex response.
2+	Normal	Slight muscle contraction with slight joint movement.
3+	Hyperreflexia	Clearly visible, brisk muscle contraction with moderate joint movement.
4+	Abnormal	Strong muscle contraction with one to three beats of clonus. Reflex spread to contralateral side may be noted.
5+	Abnormal	Strong muscle contraction with sustained clonus. Reflex spread to contralateral side may be noted.

in the threshold stimulus needed to evoke the response and a parallel decrease in the reflex latency. Not infrequently, the reflexogenous zone is extended or enlarged, and the motor response is prolonged.

Clonus is a phenomenon characterized by the rapid contraction and relaxation of agonist and antagonist muscle groups in response to a rapid stretch of one of the two muscle groups. It is most easily observed in the ankle but can be seen at the wrist and knee (patella). Clonus at the ankle can be elicited by pushing the foot briskly into dorsiflexion, thereby stretching the posterior leg muscles. The knee should be kept in slight flexion to maximize the response at the ankle. By convention, grade 4+ hyperactivity is characterized by one to three beats of clonus (unsustained), whereas grade 5+ is used to refer to a hyperactive reflex response with sustained clonus. Clonus is most commonly seen in patients with severe spasticity and is generally considered a sign of damage to the corticospinal (pyramidal) system.

Muscle stretch reflexes may also be found to be absent, but this finding is not necessarily a sign of neurologic disease. In fact, the most common cause of areflexia is poor technique on the part of the examiner. But poor technique notwithstanding, some normal people simply do not demonstrate muscle stretch reflexes. A reflex should not be designated as absent unless reinforcement is used and the examiner is convinced that the technique applied was appropriate and adequate.

Reflex responses of 1+, 2+, and 3+ are not by themselves indicative of normalcy or disease. An important finding suggestive of neurologic disease in individuals without clonus is the presence of reflex asymmetry. For example, abnormality may be suspected in a patient with a biceps brachii reflex response of 3+ on the right side and 1+ on the left side. However, based on these findings alone, the clinician will be unable to judge whether the patient is hyperreflexic on the right side or hyporeflexic on the left side. Additional information regarding other aspects of the patient's neurologic status will be required to determine which reflex response is abnormal. Symmetry is as important as reflex grade in evaluating muscle stretch reflex responses.

Several methods can be used to document muscle stretch reflex findings in the patient's permanent record. One method is to list the reflexes by name, followed by the assigned grade. Another more practical method is to indicate the reflex grade on a small stick figure that can be drawn in the patient's record. (Fig. 23).

Common Tests

Although many muscle stretch reflexes can be evaluated, only a few are routinely tested. The following section identifies the reflexes that each examiner should be able to elicit and lists the neural segments and peripheral nerves involved.

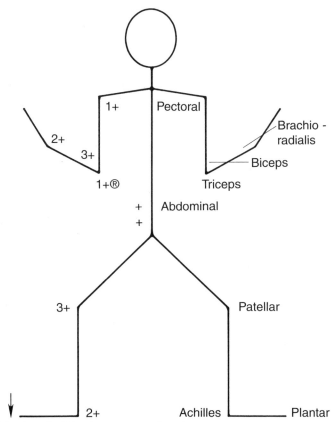

FIGURE 23. A method for documenting reflex observations in a patient's record. The names shown are those of muscle stretch reflexes and cutaneous reflexes commonly tested, and the numerical grades and symbols document reflex responses. A "+" sign for the abdominal reflexes indicates that the response was present; a minus sign indicates an absent response. The normal response to the plantar reflex is flexion of the toes, indicated by a downward-pointing arrow. An abnormal plantar reflex (Babinski sign) would be indicated by an upward-pointing arrow. "®" indicates that reinforcement was used to elicit the reflex response.

Upper Limb

Reflexes in the upper limb can be conveniently tested with the patient sitting comfortably in the bed or in a chair with a low back. The patient should be relaxed, with the arms resting comfortably in the lap. The forearms should be in the neutral position or slightly pronated.

Scapulohumeral reflex (dorsal scapular nerve, C_4–C_5).
   Percussion of the vertebral border of the scapula produces retraction (adduction) of the scapula.

Pectoral reflex (medial and lateral pectoral nerves, C_5–T_1).
Percussion of a finger pressed against the anterior axillary fold produces adduction and internal rotation of the humerus. (This may be useful when other upper limb reflexes cannot be tested.)

Deltoid reflex (axillary nerve, C_5–C_6).
Percussion of the tendon of the deltoid immediately proximal to the deltoid tubercle of the humerus produces abduction of the humerus.

Biceps brachii reflex (musculocutaneous nerve, C_5–C_6).
Percussion of the tendon of the biceps brachii in the cubital fossa produces flexion of the elbow. The response may be more clearly seen if the forearm is placed in the pronated position.

Brachioradialis reflex (radial nerve, C_5–C_6).
Percussion of the tendon of the brachioradialis immediately proximal and slightly dorsal to the styloid process of the radius produces elbow flexion and slight radial deviation or wrist extension. Wrist movement results from stretch applied to the tendons of the extensor carpi radialis longus and brevis muscles. If the forearm is placed in the pronated position, the response may include weak supination.

Triceps brachii reflex (radial nerve, C_6–C_8).
Percussion of the tendon of the triceps brachii immediately proximal to the olecranon process of the ulna produces extension of the elbow.

Finger flexor reflex (median nerve, C_6–T_1).
Percussion of the examiner's finger resting across the palmar surface of the distal phalanges of the medial four fingers produces finger flexion.

Lower Limb

Reflexes in the lower limb can be conveniently tested with the patient lying comfortably in bed or sitting upright in a firm, standard-sized chair. Restrictive bed linen and clothing should be removed so as not to impede reflex-induced movements.

Quadriceps (patellar, knee jerk) reflex (femoral nerve, L_2–L_4).
Percussion of the patellar ligament (not the tendon) produces knee extension. (*Note:* The patellar *ligament* connects the distal apex of the patella with the tibial tubercle. The patellar *tendon* courses from the proximal border of the patella to the muscle fibers of the quadriceps femoris.)

Adductor reflex (obturator nerve, L_2–L_4).
Percussion of the tendon of the adductor magnus immediately proximal to the adductor tubercle of the femur produces adduction of the thigh.

Hamstring reflex (tibial branch of sciatic nerve, L_4–S_3).
Percussion of the tendon of the semitendinosus (medial hamstring)

or long head of the biceps femoris (lateral hamstring) produces flexion of the knee. The patient should be lying prone with the knees and hips extended.

Achilles (ankle jerk) reflex (tibial nerve, L_4-S_3).
Percussion of the Achilles tendon proximal to the calcaneus produces plantar flexion of the foot. To elicit this reflex properly, it may be necessary either to maintain the knee in the extended position or to push the foot into a slight degree of dorsiflexion before percussing the tendon.

Abnormal Muscle Stretch Reflexes

The muscle stretch reflexes just described can all be elicited in the normal individual. However, several muscle stretch reflexes are not typically seen in neurologically intact individuals, but rather suggest neurologic disease. Four such abnormal reflexes are described next.

Jaw Reflex (trigeminal nerve, cranial nerve V).
The examiner depresses the patient's jaw slightly with a finger and then percusses the finger to open the jaw further. The stimulus stretches the masseter and temporalis muscles, resulting in contraction of those muscles to produce closure of the jaw. The reflex is reported as positive or present when the jaw reflexly closes and absent when no jaw movement occurs. The presence of a jaw reflex is suggestive of upper motor neuron disease or frontal lobe damage.

Snout Reflex (facial nerve, cranial nerve VII).
The examiner percusses the patient's upper lip in the midline in the region of the philtrum. The stimulus stretches muscle fibers of the orbicularis oris, producing a brief puckering or pursing of the lips. The reflex is reported as positive or present when puckering occurs and absent when no muscle response is seen. The presence of a snout reflex suggests upper motor neuron disease or frontal lobe damage.

Glabellar reflex (facial nerve, cranial nerve VII).
The examiner percusses the glabella. The stimulus stretches muscle fibers of the orbicularis oculi, producing a blinking response of the eyes. The reflex is reported as positive or present when each of several successive taps is followed by a blink response and absent when the blink response adapts after one or two taps. The presence of a glabellar reflex suggests upper motor neuron disease or frontal lobe damage.

Hoffmann's reflex (median nerve, C_6-C_8).
The examiner supports the patient's long finger at the distal interphalangeal joint, maintaining the wrist in the neutral position, the metacarpophalangeal joint in slight extension, and the interphalangeal joints in slight flexion. The examiner then flicks the distal pha-

lanx into flexion, allowing it to spring back abruptly into extension. The stimulus briefly stretches the flexor digitorum profundus muscle, which reflexly results in flexion of the thumb and index finger. The reflex is reported as positive or present when the thumb and index finger move briefly toward opposition. A positive Hoffmann reflex is suggestive of upper motor neuron disease or frontal lobe damage.

CUTANEOUS REFLEXES

Cutaneous reflexes, like muscle stretch reflexes, are normally occurring responses to stimuli that help to preserve the functional and structural integrity of the individual. The adequate stimulus for these reflexes is a strong, noxious stimulus applied to the skin. The motor response is contraction of particular muscles or muscle groups. Receptors associated with cutaneous reflexes are located in the dermal layers of the skin. The afferent limb is represented by thinly myelinated A_δ and unmyelinated C fibers, which constitute the majority of fibers in a peripheral nerve. The efferent limb and effector are motor units with alpha motor neurons located in the neural segments that receive the afferent input, or in adjacent segments. A major anatomic difference between cutaneous and muscle stretch reflexes is that cutaneous reflexes are multisynaptic in nature, whereas muscle stretch reflexes are monosynaptic. That is to say, the reflex arc for cutaneous reflexes contains at least one interneuron interposed between the afferent and efferent limbs.

In general, cutaneous reflexes are characterized by a brief contraction of skeletal muscles innervated by motor neurons located in the same segments that receive the afferent input. However, this characteristic is partly related to the stimulus employed. If the stimulus is too weak, it may fail to elicit a response at all. If the stimulus is too strong, it may elicit an exaggerated response indicating the spread of nerve impulses to other segments of the neuraxis, including the brainstem and forebrain. The stronger or more noxious the stimulus, the more likely it is that the afferent barrage will spread to adjacent segments and produce a more widespread effect. Such an exaggerated response is referred to as a *withdrawal reflex*. The cutaneous reflexes with which you should be familiar are described next.

Abdominal Reflexes

The abdominal reflexes are elicited by scratching the skin of the anterior abdominal wall with a sharp object. The stimulus should be directed from lateral to medial, keeping the stimulus within a single dermatome on one side of the abdomen. The normal response is deviation of the umbilicus toward the stimulus. The stimulus should not be delivered from medial to lateral, because this motion might result in a mechanical displacement of the umbilicus away from the midline, thereby obscuring the normal response. Each side of the abdomen should be tested separately. When the umbilicus moves in the direction of the applied stimulus, the reflex is documented as present or positive. A method for documenting abdominal reflex responses on the stick figure used to record muscle stretch reflexes is illustrated in Figure 23.

The abdominal reflexes are helpful in evaluating the integrity of spinal segments T-6–L-1. Stimuli applied in the hypochondriac regions of the abdomen (above the level of the umbilicus) produce umbilical deviation in a superolateral direction and involve spinal segments T-6–T-9. Stimuli applied in the ilioinguinal region (below the level of the umbilicus) produce umbilical deviation in an inferolateral direction and involve spinal segments T-11–L-1. Stimulation delivered at the level of the umbilicus produces lateral deviation of the umbilicus, which is mediated by afferent and efferent fibers associated with the T-10 segment of the spinal cord.

The abdominal reflexes can be elicited in most neurologically intact individuals. They may be absent or difficult to elicit in obese individuals or women in the late stages of pregnancy. Loss of abdominal reflexes is most often a sign of corticospinal (pyramidal) system disease. A possible explanation for this finding is that a substantial number of corticospinal axons originate from neurons in the anterior gyri of the parietal lobe (areas 1, 2, 3, and 5), and these cells are thought to influence interneurons and ascending tract cells located in the dorsal horn of the spinal cord. Cortically originating influences, probably excitatory in nature, may help to keep spinal interneurons and lower motor neurons near threshold. When the excitatory effect of these descending corticospinal axons is lost, interneurons and lower motor neurons may be moved sufficiently away from threshold (hyperpolarized) that cutaneous stimuli arriving by way of segmental afferent fibers are insufficient to evoke the normal cutaneous reflex response. Loss of the abdominal reflexes, particularly on one side only, is frequently seen in patients who have suffered a stroke and is considered an early sign of damage to the corticospinal (pyramidal) system.

Cremasteric Reflex

The cremasteric reflex is characterized by elevation of the testicle in response to stroking of the skin of the proximal and medial part of the thigh. The afferent limb is derived from cutaneous branches of the ilioinguinal nerve supplying the skin of the thigh adjacent to the scrotum. The efferent limb is the genital branch of the genitofemoral nerve, which provides motor innervation to the cremaster muscle. The reflex involves the

L-1 and L-2 segments of the spinal cord and is normally present in neurologically intact individuals. It may be lost in patients who sustain injuries involving lumbosacral segments of the spinal cord or who have lesions involving the axons of the corticospinal (pyramidal) system.

Bulbocavernosus Reflex

The bulbocavernosus reflex is characterized by a palpable contraction of the bulbospongiosus muscle at the base of the penis in response to pinching the glans penis. The reflex is mediated by afferent and efferent fibers, both carried in the pudendal nerve. The reflex is normally present in the neurologically intact individual and involves spinal cord levels S-2–4. It may be lost in patients who sustain injuries involving the conus medullaris or sacral spinal roots, or who have lesions involving the axons of the corticospinal (pyramidal) system.

Anal Sphincter Reflex

The anal sphincter reflex is characterized by contraction of the external anal sphincter in response to scratching the perianal skin. The afferent and efferent limbs of the reflex are carried in the pudendal nerve and involve the S-2–4 segments of the spinal cord. The reflex is normally present in neurologically intact individuals. It may be lost in patients who sustain injuries involving the conus medullaris or who have lesions involving the axons of the corticospinal (pyramidal) system.

Plantar Reflex

The plantar reflex is one of the most useful and frequently tested reflexes in clinical neurology. The afferent limb of the reflex is the tibial nerve (lateral and medial plantar branches) and involves the S-1 and S-2 segments of the spinal cord. The efferent limb is also the tibial nerve, with axons originating from alpha motor neurons located in L-5–S-2 spinal segments. The normal reflex response in the adult is plantar flexion of the toes produced by contraction of the flexor digitorum longus, flexor hallucis longus, and lumbrical muscles of the foot. The normal response may take up to half a second to develop and appear.

Proper technique is essential if the response to stimulation is to be interpreted correctly. If the stimulus is too weak, too brief, or inadequate in some other way, no response may be obtained, and the examiner may conclude that disease is present when in fact it is not. If the stimulus is too strong, the response elicited might represent a withdrawal phenomenon and again mislead the examiner. The correct stimulus must be appropriate in location, intensity, and duration.

The stimulus should be delivered with an object that produces a noxious or unpleasant, but not frankly painful, sensation. The stimulus should be delivered on the sole of the foot in a sweeping motion beginning at the calcaneus, proceeding distally over the shaft of the fifth metatarsal, then turning medially across the metatarsal heads. The stimulus should be even in pressure and require approximately one full second to deliver. An adequate stimulus will allow for both the temporal and spatial summation of afferent impulses necessary to evoke the response. Stimulation that is delivered too quickly or that does not cover the full territory may be inadequate and subthreshold.

In addition to an adequate stimulus, other conditions must be present for proper testing of this reflex response. The patient's knee should be fully extended. The response may be absent if the knee is flexed. Other factors that can influence the response include foot temperature, thickness of the plantar calluses, and the general sensitivity of the skin of the sole of the foot. If the foot is cold, the reflex response may be reduced in amplitude. Thick plantar calluses can make the response difficult to elicit or cause the reflex to be absent. Individuals with normally hypersensitive feet may demonstrate an exaggerated response to plantar stimulation or possibly exhibit a withdrawal response that can easily fool the unwary examiner. For mechanical reasons, the plantar response may be difficult to obtain in patients with pes cavus. Patients with peripheral neuropathy involving the tibial nerve may have absent or reduced plantar responses.

The proper way to report the response to plantar stimulation is to describe what occurs simply and completely. The description of the normal response should clearly indicate that the toes were downgoing. A method for documenting the normal plantar response using the stick figure is illustrated in Figure 23.

Because some patients have hypersensitive feet, it may be necessary to use an alternative form of stimulation to elicit the plantar reflex. Noxious stimulation delivered in a proximal-to-distal direction along the tibial crest (Oppenheim) or along the lateral edge of the foot (Chaddock) will produce downgoing toes in the neurologically intact individual. Alternatively, noxious squeezing of the calf muscles (Gordon) or the Achilles tendon (Schaefer) will have the same result. Again, movement of the toes should be precisely described in the patient's record.

Abnormal Plantar Responses

In patients with neurologic damage involving the corticospinal (pyramidal) system, stimulation of the plantar surface of the foot, or any of the alternative forms of stimulation just described, may result in dorsiflexion of the great toe and fanning (abduction) of the lateral four toes. This abnormal response to plantar stimulation is commonly referred to as the *Babin-*

ski reflex or *response*. It is an example of a pathologic cutaneous (superficial) reflex. The afferent limb of this abnormal reflex response is the tibial nerve, as described previously, but the motor response is mediated by axons carried in both the peroneal nerve (deep peroneal branch) and the tibial nerve (lateral plantar branch). Impulse transmission in the peroneal nerve leads to contraction of the extensor hallucis longus, which causes extension of the great toe, and impulse transmission in the tibial nerve excites the abductor digiti minimi and dorsal interossei muscles, which cause abduction (fanning) of the toes.

The exact mechanism whereby plantar stimulation produces downgoing toes in the normal individual but an upgoing great toe with fanning of the other toes in patients with corticospinal damage is unclear, although a rational explanation can be offered. In the neurologically intact individual, cutaneous stimulation produces contraction of muscles innervated by neurons located in the same spinal segments. The abdominal reflex is an example of this phenomenon. In the lower limb, stimulation of the plantar surface of the foot produces a reflex contraction of the toe and foot flexors as part of the placing reaction necessary to counteract the force of gravity while standing. A similar neurologic mechanism exists in the forelimbs of quadripedal animals. Cortical control over these reflex mechanisms is mediated by corticospinal axons coursing through the cerebral peduncle, medullary pyramid, and lateral corticospinal tract. These axons provide excitatory influences on predominantly *flexor* motor neuron pools innervating predominantly *distal* muscle groups. If these excitatory influences are lost, as would be the case when the corticospinal system is damaged, distal flexor lower motor neuron pools would be brought slightly, but nonetheless significantly, away from threshold (hyperpolarized). Under these conditions, a barrage of afferent impulses produced by a slowly moving noxious stimulus applied to the plantar surface of the foot might be inadequate to excite the hyperpolarized flexor motor neurons but sufficient to activate *extensor* lower motor neuron pools that were not affected in any appreciable way by the lesion. The Babinski response may therefore reflect a relative shift in the effect of afferent nerve impulses from flexor motor neuron pools to extensor motor neuron pools. The motor response may reflect the loss of excitation of flexor motor neurons rather than a loss of inhibition of extensor motor neurons, as is commonly suggested.

The term Babinski reflex or response is firmly entrenched in the neurologic vocabulary but is frequently misused in day-to-day conversation. The Babinski response, which consists of dorsiflexion of the great toe and fanning of the lateral four toes following strong stimulation delivered to the plantar surface of the foot, is either *present* or *absent*. Upgoing toes in response to plantar stimulation mean that the response is present; downgoing toes mean the response is absent. It is incorrect to say that the response is positive when the toes extend (go up) and negative when the toes flex (go down). Students have been confused about this matter in the past and are likely to be confused about it in the future. The best way to report the findings of the plantar, Oppenheim, Chaddock, Gordon, or Schaefer reflex is simply to indicate whether the toes go up or down in response to stimulation.

An abnormal plantar reflex (upgoing toes) suggests corticospinal (pyramidal) system damage. Abnormal cutaneous reflex responses can also be elicited from the upper limb. The *palmomental reflex*, contraction of the mentalis muscle in response to tactile stimulation of the palm of the hand, is not seen in neurologically intact individuals but may be seen in patients with damage to the frontal lobe or corticospinal system. Similarly, the *palmar grasp reflex*, flexion of the fingers and thumb in response to tactile stimulation of the palm, may be seen in patients suffering from diseases involving the frontal lobe or corticospinal system. These two pathologic reflexes are particularly useful in that they are present in disease states but absent in the normal individual.

SUMMARY

Reflex testing can provide the examiner with useful information regarding the functional integrity of specific components of both the peripheral and the central nervous systems. In general, muscle stretch reflexes are depressed or absent in patients with peripheral nerve disease and increased in patients with lesions involving central nervous system structures. Similarly, muscle stretch reflexes are typically reduced or absent in patients with lower motor neuron disease, but increased in patients with disease involving upper motor neurons.

In contrast, cutaneous reflexes are generally lost in patients with both peripheral and central nervous system disease. Pathologic reflexes may be elicited in patients with disease or injury involving central nervous system structures. Finally, it is important to bear in mind that the most persuasive indicator of neurologic disease with regard to muscle stretch reflexes and cutaneous reflexes is side-to-side asymmetry.

CHAPTER 7

SENSORY SYSTEMS

The sensory systems are composed of both neural and non-neural structures that function to provide us with an awareness of the environment in which we live. Traditionally, we recognize an exteroceptive sense, having to do with the environment outside the body; an enteroceptive sense, concerned with the visceral or internal structures of the body; and a proprioceptive sense, an awareness of the relative position of the body or various body parts in space. Kinesthesia is a sense closely related to proprioception, which refers specifically to awareness of the movement of body parts. Normal sensory function can be thought of as being composed of four distinct processes: sensory transduction, impulse transmission, perception, and sensory interpretation.

FUNCTIONAL ANATOMY

Sensory transduction is the process whereby stimuli or energy applied to the body results in the generation of action potentials in peripheral nerves. Sensory transduction is achieved either by specialized receptors located in visceral and somatic structures, or directly in peripheral nerve fibers without specialized receptors, which are sensitive to changes in the microenvironment in which they are located. Sensory receptors transduce or convert a particular form of energy into nerve impulses, which are transmitted toward the central nervous system (CNS).

Impulse transmission is the process whereby information about the environment in the form of action potentials is brought to the CNS and distributed to regions where, among other functions, perception and interpretation occur. Afferent nerve cells with cell bodies located in dorsal root ganglia and cranial nerve sensory ganglia transmit nerve impulses from the periphery to the CNS. Within the CNS, several ascending pathways are involved in distributing nerve impulses to specific areas of the brain important in perception and interpretation.

Perception is the phenomenon of experiencing the environment and changes in it. Specific nuclei of the dorsal thalamus and gyri of the cerebral hemispheres are thought to be involved in sensory perception. In humans, the primary sensory cortex is the postcentral gyrus of the parietal lobe. This region of cortex is somatotopically organized, which suggests that it may be important for localizing stimuli affecting receptor structures in different areas of the body.

Sensory interpretation is a process in which meaning and significance are assigned to the perceived attributes of an event or object in the environment. It results in recognition of the event or object and is based on some previous experience with it. Sensory interpretation is a higher cortical function and involves areas of the cerebral cortex commonly referred to as *association cortices*. The recognition or interpretation of tactile stimuli involves the association cortex of the parietal lobe.

The anatomic and functional organization of the sensory systems are reviewed briefly in this chapter. Sensory functions associated with cranial nerves were described previously and are not reviewed here. This discussion focuses on somatic sensory functions mediated by spinal nerves and pathways, functions that are routinely evaluated in the sensory part of the neurologic examination.

Sensory receptors located in the skin and other somatic structures are classified in a number of ways. For our purposes, only four characteristics of sensory receptors need to be considered: morphology, modality, threshold, and adaptation rate.

Morphologically, the peripheral end of an afferent nerve fiber can be described as being encapsulated or unencapsulated. *Encapsulated* nerve fibers are characterized by specialized sensory endings at their distal end. In the past, these specialized receptor endings were referred to by their eponyms (i.e., Ruffini, Merkel, Meissner, Krause, Pacinian), but these names are gradually being replaced by more functional and informative terms. *Unencapsulated* nerve endings lack a specialized structure for energy transduction. Such fibers are described as having free nerve endings. More peripheral nerve fibers in the skin have free nerve endings than have encapsulated endings.

Modality refers to the type of energy to which a receptor preferentially responds. For the purpose of the neurologic examination, two distinct receptor subtypes found in the skin should be noted: mechanoreceptors and thermoreceptors. *Mechanoreceptors* respond maximally and most sensitively to mechanical energy, usually in the form of tissue distortion or stretch. *Thermoreceptors* respond to thermal energy applied to the body. Some receptors in the skin respond to both mechanical and thermal stimuli. These are referred to as *polymodal* receptors.

Threshold refers to the amount of energy needed to activate the receptor and induce the centripetal transmission of an action potential in the afferent fiber with which the receptor is associated. Low-threshold receptors respond to low levels of applied energy; high-threshold receptors require a substantial amount of energy to respond. High-threshold receptors that respond most vigorously to intense, tissue-damaging amounts of energy are sometimes referred to as *nociceptors*. Clinically and experimentally, we recognize several classes of nociceptors, including mechanonociceptors, thermonociceptors, and polymodal nociceptors.

Adaptation is a process in which a receptor becomes less sensitive or responsive to a stimulus or form of energy to which it normally responds. *Adaptation rate* refers to the speed at which a receptor stops firing or reduces its firing rate after the application of a particular stimulus. *Slowly adapting* receptors do not demonstrate adaptation (i.e., they continue to respond in a stable way so long as the stimulus is being applied). Receptors that reduce their firing rate fairly quickly over time in response to a sustained stimulus are referred to as *rapidly adapting*. A special type of receptor in the skin, the pacinian corpuscle, adapts almost immediately after firing and is referred to as a *very rapidly adapting* receptor.

Sensory receptors with diverse characteristics are essential for normal living. As we will see, a knowledge of these characteristics is crucial to an understanding of why particular stimuli are used in the sensory examination. Each is more or less specific to certain anatomic and functional systems.

The transmission of nerve impulses from the receptor in the periphery to the CNS occurs along the axons of afferent nerve cells derived from the neural crest. The cell bodies of these neurons compose segmental dorsal root ganglia and are pseudounipolar in structure. The central processes of dorsal root ganglion cells constitute the dorsal roots and enter the spinal cord along the dorsolateral fissure in a region frequently referred to as the *dorsal root entry zone* (DREZ). The peripheral processes of spinal afferent neurons combine to form segmental spinal nerves, which may intermingle further in plexuses (i.e., brachial or lumbosacral) to form specific peripheral nerves.

Dorsal root ganglion cells and their peripheral processes vary in size. The more thickly myelinated afferent fibers transmit nerve impulses to the spinal cord more rapidly than do the thinly myelinated and nonmyelinated fibers. Table 12 identifies different classes of spinal afferent fibers and gives information about their diameter, conduction velocity, and function.

Transmission of nerve impulses from the dorsal root ganglion to the spinal cord occurs along axons that form the dorsal roots. As each root

TABLE 12 *Classification of Peripheral Afferent Nerve Fibers*

Fiber Type	Diameter (μm)	Conduction Velocity (m/sec)	Function
Ia	15–20	70–120	Muscle spindles
Ib	15–20	70–120	Tendon organs
II, A_β	5–20	30–70	Muscle spindles Low-threshold mechanoreceptors
A_δ	2–5	12–30	Thermoreceptors High-threshold mechanoreceptors Nociceptors
C	0.5–1	0.5–2	Thermoreceptors High-threshold mechanoreceptors Nociceptors

approaches the spinal cord, it further divides into a series of longitudinally oriented rootlets that penetrate the pial surface in the region of the dorsolateral fissure. The axons within each rootlet segregate in the region of the DREZ in such a way that the more thickly myelinated fibers enter the cord slightly medial to the more thinly myelinated and unmyelinated axons (Fig. 24).

Most of the axons entering the spinal cord via the dorsal root termi-

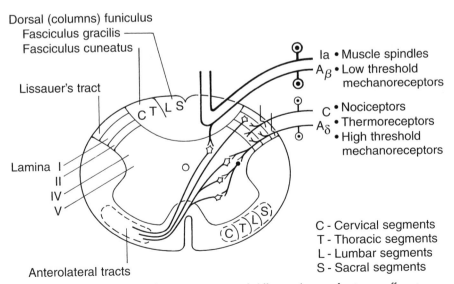

FIGURE 24. The spinal cord termination sites of different classes of primary afferent nerve fibers.

nate in the ipsilateral dorsal horn. Immediately on entering the DREZ, thinly myelinated A_δ and C fibers divide into ascending and descending branches, which occupy the dorsolateral fasciculus, more commonly known as Lissauer's tract. Primary afferent axons in Lissauer's tract extend for two to three segments in both directions before terminating in the superficial laminae of the dorsal horn. As a result, nerve impulses entering the spinal cord at a particular segment can influence dorsal horn neurons located at several adjacent levels. In physiologic terms, the process is referred to as *divergence.*

The more thickly myelinated afferent fibers enter the spinal cord somewhat medially, near the border between the dorsal horn and the dorsal funiculus. Within the spinal cord, these axons divide into several branches. One terminates in the nucleus proprius of the dorsal horn and another occupies a somatotopically organized position in the dorsal funiculus (see Fig. 24).

Some clinically useful generalizations can be made at this time regarding the functional relationship between certain sensory receptors and particular classes of primary afferent fibers. In general, low-threshold, rapidly adapting, encapsulated receptors tend to be associated with thickly myelinated afferent fibers, whereas high-threshold, slowly adapting, unencapsulated receptors, including nociceptors and thermoreceptors, tend to be associated with thinly myelinated and unmyelinated afferent nerve fibers. These general concepts serve as the bases for selecting particular stimuli for use in the sensory portion of the neurologic examination.

Within the spinal cord, nerve impulses are transmitted to more rostral levels of the neuraxis by way of two major ascending pathways, the anterolateral system (ALS) and the dorsal column–medial lemniscus system (DC-ML). The anatomic organization and function of each of these ascending systems is briefly reviewed.

Anterolateral System

The ALS is composed of several ascending tracts that occupy a position in the anterolateral white matter of the spinal cord. These fibers originate in cells on the contralateral side of the spinal cord, in the dorsal, intermediate, and ventral horns. The axons cross the midline in the anterior white commissure before accumulating in the anterolateral white matter (see Fig. 24). The axons that form the anterolateral tracts are somatotopically organized. Those that subserve sacral and lumbar segments are dorsolateral to those that subserve thoracic and cervical levels. A somatotopic organization is retained throughout the brainstem, where the term *spinal lemniscus* is used to refer to these axons.

For our purposes, the most important of the ascending pathways that make up the ALS are the spinothalamic, spinoreticular, and spinotectal tracts.

The *spinothalamic tract*, as the name implies, terminates in particular nuclei of the dorsal thalamus. These nuclei include the ventral posterolateral (VPL), intralaminar, and dorsomedial (DM) nuclei (Fig. 25). Some spinothalamic projections are also reported to terminate in the hypothalamus, thereby providing a substrate for autonomic and visceral reactions that are sometimes seen in association with noxious or unpleasant sensory stimuli.

Thalamocortical projections from each of these dorsal thalamic nuclei differ and are thought to be important in different aspects of the sensory experience. Nerve cells in the VPL nucleus are somatotopically organized and are the origin of a somatotopically organized projection through the posterior limb of the internal capsule to the postcentral gyrus (areas 3, 1, 2 of Brodmann) (Fig. 26). Experimental and clinical evidence has shown that the medial (interhemispheric) surface of the postcentral gyrus receives information from sacral and lumbar levels, whereas the dorsal and dorsolateral surfaces receive information from thoracic and cervical spinal levels. Cortical areas subserving the lower limb receive arterial blood by way of branches of the anterior cerebral artery, whereas areas associated with sensation from the upper limb are perfused by branches of the middle cerebral artery. Knowledge of this pattern of vascular anatomy can be useful in evaluating patients with suspected cerebral vascular disease involving the carotid circulation.

Impulse transmission in this neuronal system terminating in the postcentral gyrus is thought to be important in localizing the site of an applied stimulus and in the sensory-discriminative aspects of pain. Impulse transmission from the intralaminar nuclei and the DM nucleus is more widely distributed, particularly to cortical areas in the frontal lobe. These areas of the brain are thought to be important in value judgments regarding sensory experiences, complex reactions to sensory stimulation, and in motivational and affective responses to noxious or painful experiences.

Spinoreticular projections coursing through the anterolateral tracts and spinal lemniscus terminate in nuclei scattered throughout the reticular formation of the brainstem (see Fig. 25). These nuclei in turn participate in a number of functions, three of which are pertinent to our understanding of normal neurologic function and the neurologic examination.

First, ascending projections originating in the brainstem reticular formation exert an excitatory effect on the cerebral cortex, mediated through the thalamus. Activity in this ascending reticular activating system (ARAS) is essential to maintenance of the conscious state. As activity in the ARAS is depressed, so is level of consciousness. We use this knowledge when we apply noxious sensory stimuli in an effort to arouse a co-

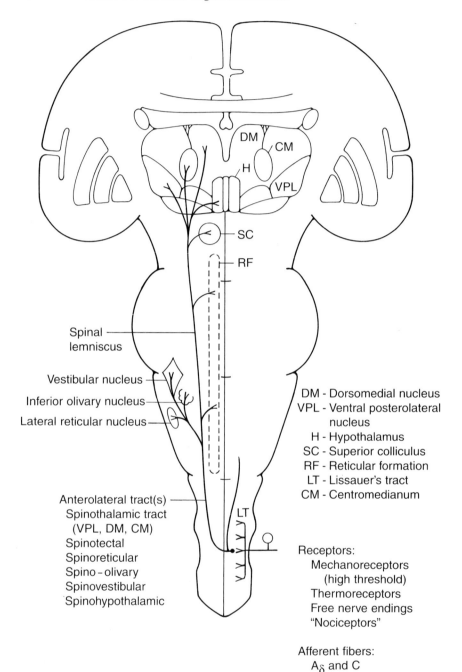

DM - Dorsomedial nucleus
VPL - Ventral posterolateral
      nucleus
H - Hypothalamus
SC - Superior colliculus
RF - Reticular formation
LT - Lissauer's tract
CM - Centromedianum

Receptors:
  Mechanoreceptors
    (high threshold)
  Thermoreceptors
  Free nerve endings
    "Nociceptors"

Afferent fibers:
  A_δ and C

FIGURE 25. Brainstem and forebrain nuclei that receive afferent input from axons of the anterolateral system. (Modified from Haines, DE: *Neuroanatomy: An Atlas of Structures, Sections, and Systems,* ed 3. Urban & Schwartzenberg, Baltimore and Munich, 1991, with permission.)

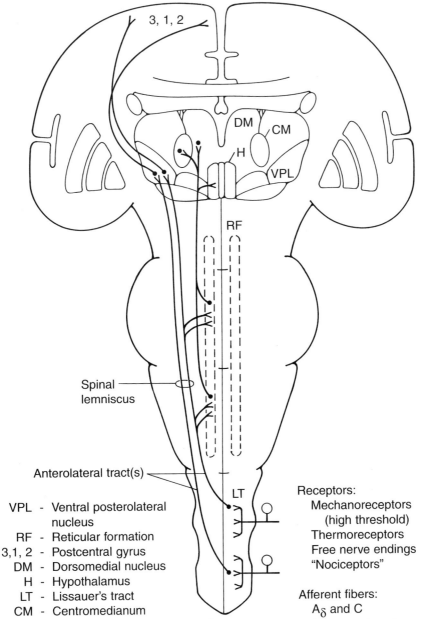

FIGURE 26. The course and termination of major components of the anterolateral system. (Modified from Haines, DE: *Neuroanatomy: An Atlas of Structures, Sections, and Systems*, ed 3. Urban & Schwartzenberg, Baltimore and Munich, 1991, with permission.)

matose or stuporous patient. When we apply a noxious stimulus, we are increasing neural activity in spinoreticular, reticulothalamic, and thalamocortical pathways in an effort to raise the level of consciousness.

Second, descending projections from the brainstem reticular formation to autonomic and somatic motor neurons in the spinal cord activate defense systems to protect the individual from continuing exteroceptive insult. In this sense, spinoreticular projections activate moderately complex, automatic behaviors that are part of self-protective defensive mechanisms.

Third, descending projections from specific nuclear regions of the brainstem reticular formation exert an inhibitory influence on the very ascending tract cells that excited them in the first place. Recent studies have identified a functionally distinct group of neurons in the mesencephalic periaqueductal gray and the pontine and medullary raphe that are involved in this primitive inhibitory system. Some of the neurons in this system may be involved in the mediation of opioid analgesia.

The final pathway to consider in this brief review of the ALS is the spinotectal tract. The axons of this tract lie intermixed with those of the spinothalamic and spinoreticular tracts in the spinal cord and brainstem. At the level of the midbrain, spinotectal axons terminate in the deeper layers of the superior colliculus (see Fig. 25). Nerve cells of the superior colliculus that receive spinal input are the origin of axons that descend through the brainstem and enter the spinal cord as the tectospinal tract. Tectal projections to the brainstem (tectobulbar) are distributed to the extraocular nuclei. The pathway helps mediate eye movements to bring a stimulated area of skin into the visual field. In the spinal cord, tectospinal fibers terminate on interneurons and lower motor neurons that innervate muscles that support the neck and move the head. Activity in this pathway also helps to bring stimulated areas into view by producing appropriate movements of the head. The spinotectal component of the ALS can therefore be viewed as the ascending portion of a neural system that can be used to orient the position of the eyes in the skull and the head on the trunk in response to stimulation of the skin.

Dorsal Column–Medial Lemniscus System

The dorsal column–medial lemniscus system is a phylogenetically newer ascending pathway. The dorsal columns (dorsal funiculi) are composed of two smaller fasciculi: the fasciculus gracilis and the more laterally located fasciculus cuneatus (see Fig. 24). The fasciculus gracilis is composed of the central processes of large dorsal root ganglion cells subserving sacral, lumbar, and lower thoracic spinal segments of the ipsilateral side. The cell bodies of axons forming the fasciculus cuneatus are located in dorsal root ganglia associated with upper thoracic and cervical levels of the spinal cord (Fig. 27). The dorsal columns are somatotopically orga-

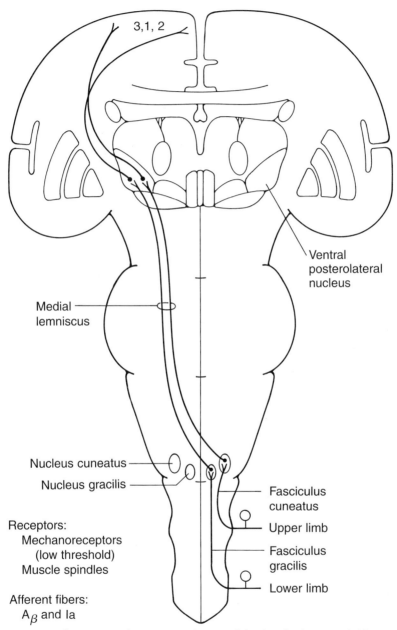

FIGURE 27. The course and termination of axons of the dorsal column–medial lemniscus system. 3, 1, 2 = Postcentral gyrus. (Modified from Haines, DE: *Neuroanatomy: An Atlas of Structures, Sections, and Systems*, ed 3. Urban & Schwartzenberg, Baltimore and Munich, 1991, with permission.)

nized, with fibers subserving sacral segments being most medial and those transmitting impulses from cervical levels being most lateral (see Fig. 24).

The axons in the fasciculus gracilis and cuneatus terminate at the level of the caudal medulla oblongata, in the nucleus gracilis and nucleus cuneatus, respectively. Nerve cells in these two nuclei are the origin of axons that cross the midline in a rostroventral trajectory and assume a position in the medulla immediately dorsal to the medullary pyramid. The crossed axons of these nuclei form a somatotopically organized bundle of fibers referred to as the medial lemniscus. The fibers of the medial lemniscus continue rostrally to terminate in the VPL nucleus of the thalamus (see Fig. 27). From the VPL nucleus, nerve impulses are transmitted to the postcentral gyrus (areas 3, 1, 2) by way of thalamocortical projections occupying the posterior limb of the internal capsule. The dorsal column–medial lemniscus system is somatotopically organized throughout its course, making it ideally suited for localizing stimuli applied to discrete regions of the body.

Perception of a stimulus implies only that it is felt or experienced. Some authors argue that perception is a thalamic function, although the specific contribution of particular thalamic nuclei to sensory experience remains uncertain. Other authors suggest that some degree of stimulus localization is required to confidently assess perception. Under this operating definition, both the VPL and the postcentral gyrus must be functionally intact for normal perception to occur. Experimental and clinical evidence has not yet completely resolved this issue, but it is clear that disease or injuries involving these specific cortical, nuclear, and white-matter areas produce definable perceptual deficits involving somatotopically appropriate areas of the body.

Sensory interpretation is a process whereby recognition or meaning is attributed to perceived stimuli. With regard to cutaneous sensory stimuli, this process includes several related functions, including the ability to identify a stimulus based on its tactile characteristics. Identifying objects by touch (stereognosis), recognizing numbers or letters written on the skin (graphesthesia), and differentiating between different weights (barognosis) are cortical functions involving sensory association cortices of the parietal lobe. Patients with focal disease involving these cortices alone present with fascinating deficits of recognition even though they are able to perceive tactile stimuli.

The anatomic organization of different components of the peripheral nervous system must be understood if the examiner is to correctly identify and localize disease processes affecting these structures. An adequate knowledge of peripheral neuroanatomy also is essential. The reader must become familiar with the cutaneous distribution of both segmentally derived sensory fibers (dermatomes) and postplexus peripheral nerves. Figures 28 and 29 illustrate regions of the body innervated by particular segmental or peripheral nerves.

CLINICAL EXAMINATIONS

Many techniques can be used to assess the integrity of the somatic sensory systems. Based on the preceding discussion of the neuroanatomic organization of the sensory systems, I will, for the sake of convenience, divide these clinical tests into three related yet distinct groups: those that assess primarily the integrity of the anterolateral system, those that assess primarily the integrity of the dorsal column–medial lemniscus system, and those that assess cortical sensory function. Specific sensory tests that will be considered within each category are listed in Table 13.

It is important to point out that the test procedures described in each category do not necessarily induce transmission of nerve impulses solely in that particular ascending tract system. Rather, the distinction between

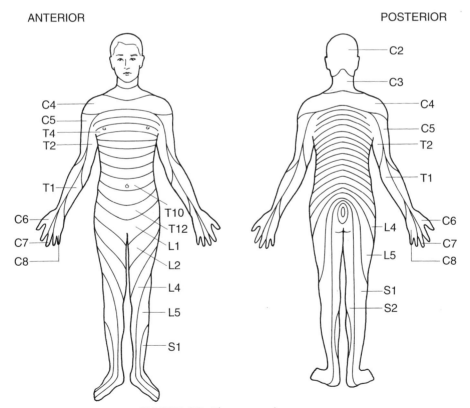

FIGURE 28. The sensory dermatomes.

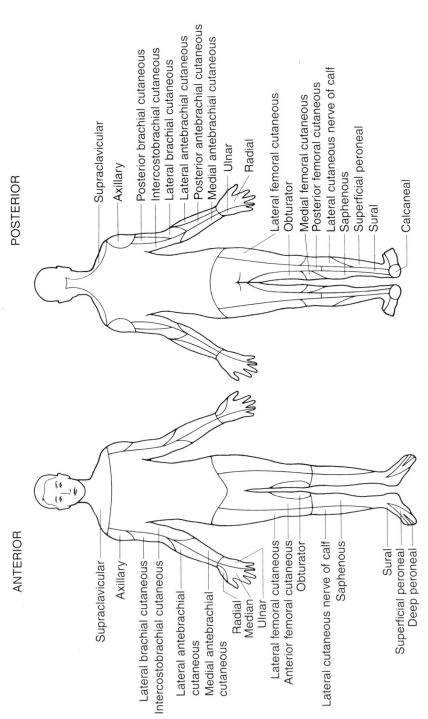

FIGURE 29. The sensory distribution of peripheral cutaneous nerves.

POSTERIOR

Supraclavicular
Axillary
Posterior brachial cutaneous
Intercostobrachial cutaneous
Lateral brachial cutaneous
Lateral antebrachial cutaneous
Posterior antebrachial cutaneous
Medial antebrachial cutaneous
Ulnar
Radial

Lateral femoral cutaneous
Obturator
Medial femoral cutaneous
Posterior femoral cutaneous
Lateral cutaneous nerve of calf
Saphenous
Superficial peroneal
Sural

Calcaneal

ANTERIOR

Supraclavicular
Axillary
Lateral brachial cutaneous
Intercostobrachial cutaneous
Lateral antebrachial cutaneous
Medial antebrachial cutaneous
Radial
Median
Ulnar
Lateral femoral cutaneous
Anterior femoral cutaneous
Obturator
Lateral cutaneous nerve of calf
Saphenous
Sural
Superficial peroneal
Deep peroneal

TABLE 13 *Classification of Clinical Tests of Sensory Function*

Functional System	Clinical Tests
Anterolateral systems	Pin prick Thermal sense Deep pain
Dorsal column—Medial lemniscus	Light touch Vibratory sense Position sense
Cortical sensory function	Traced figure identification Object identification Double simultaneous stimulation

these anatomically separate systems is based on clinical observations relating measurable clinical deficits to known neuropathology involving these systems.

By convention, sensory function tests are performed late in the neurologic examination, a situation with both advantages and disadvantages. One advantage is that by this time the clinician should have a good idea of whether the patient has a sensory deficit. If no sensory deficit is evident, a simple screening test of sensory function may be all that is necessary to ensure a complete neurologic evaluation. If sensory impairment is suspected, the clinician should have a fairly good understanding of its nature, location, and probable cause, knowledge that will aid and guide the examiner in acquiring a more precise and complete impression of the sensory abnormality. An important disadvantage, however, which is frequently overlooked, is that tests of sensory function require concentration and cooperation on the part of both the examiner and the patient. Test results are not likely to be accurate or reliable if the patient is fatigued, inattentive, distracted, or simply unable to cooperate fully for one reason or another. There is no point in performing tests of sensory function if the patient is tired. It is better to stop the examination and resume at another time.

During preparations to perform sensory function tests, the patient should be made as comfortable as possible. It is important that the examiner explain exactly what he or she intends to do to the patient and what the patient is expected to do in response. Because the tests involve the application of different types of sensory stimuli, the patient should be given the opportunity to experience each stimulus in a normal way so that he or she will be able to recognize different or abnormal sensory experiences if they can be elicited. Keep in mind that the sensory examination is the most subjective part of the neurologic evaluation, and the patient must be able to make sometimes subtle judgments about the characteristics of a sensory experience.

A variety of stimuli have been devised for use in sensory testing. Most have been chosen because they theoretically or preferentially excite a particular type of receptor in the skin or induce impulse transmission in a certain class of afferent nerve fibers. Stimuli used in clinical testing are more closely related to the receptors they activate than they are to the ascending pathways that mediate their effects.

It is worth repeating a concept developed earlier in this book regarding the relationship between specific neuroanatomic structures and neurologic function. Sensory and motor functions lost or impaired as a result of damage to specific neurologic structures should not necessarily be attributed to those damaged structures. Rather, retained but abnormal sensory and motor functions reflect neuronal activity involving the remaining, anatomically intact neural structures to effect neurologic function without the influence of the damaged structures. When we draw conclusions based on an interpretation of the results of sensory tests, we are making inferences about the location or nature of an injury or disease process based on retained sensory function. We do not assign function to a particular sensory system or component of a sensory system that we believe has been damaged. With this in mind, we now consider specific techniques and procedures that when properly performed can be useful in drawing inferences about the location and nature of particular nervous system afflictions.

The nature and characteristics of different sensory abnormalities vary greatly and are related to a number of factors. Two important alterations in sensory experience that should be sought are frank changes in the sensory characteristics of a stimulus and perceptual experiences of the same stimulus that are different in similar skin areas on the two sides of the body. Side-to-side differences in sensory experience generally suggest unilateral disease affecting peripheral or central nervous system structures. Note, however, that some peripheral nerve afflictions, particularly those that are metabolic in nature, may affect both sides equally.

Assessment of the Anterolateral System

Pin Testing

The ability to perceive noxious stimulation is part of an important protective mechanism. The sharp point of a safety pin can be used to deliver noxious stimulation for testing purposes. Pressing the sharp point of a pin against the skin is thought to activate high-threshold, slowly adapting nerve endings associated with thinly myelinated (A_δ) and unmyelinated (C) peripheral nerve fibers. Nerve impulses transmitted to the CNS along these fibers are believed to be transmitted to higher levels by way of the anterolateral tracts. Perception of noxious pin stimulation is thought to require thalamic neurons, with the ability to localize the stimulus being a function of neurons in the postcentral gyrus.

The patient should be made comfortable in either the sitting or lying position. Areas of skin to be tested should be unclothed and easily accessible to the examiner. Sensory testing cannot be adequately performed through clothing. The patient should be instructed to close his or her eyes and keep them closed while the tests are being performed.

The sharp end of a clean safety pin that has not been previously used with another patient can be used to provide stimulation. The examiner should instruct the patient to respond by saying "sharp" or "dull" immediately on feeling the stimulus. It is important for the examiner to provide the patient with an experience that fairly represents the sensation of both sharp and dull. The point of the pin can be used to represent sharp, and the blunted clasp of the pin can be used to represent dull. The examiner should apply each of these stimuli to an area of the skin that has normal sensation so that the patient has a good and unequivocal basis for making a judgment as to whether a sensation is sharp or dull. The examiner must be certain before testing begins that the patient can distinguish sharp from dull.

The test is performed by applying the sharp end of the pin to the patient's skin for a brief instant with a pressure that is sufficient to indent but not puncture the skin. Theoretically, this stimulus should be adequate to activate nociceptive receptor endings and result in the transmission of action potentials along A_δ and C fibers. The patient should be instructed to respond immediately if and when the pin is felt. If a sensory deficit is suspected, it is generally better to begin testing in the area of the deficit and to move gradually toward areas of skin where sensation is presumed to be normal. In this way, the patient is more likely to detect a change in the perceptual characteristics of the stimulus when it occurs.

The examiner must carefully and thoroughly identify areas of sensory abnormality. It is frequently helpful to mark the border between normal and abnormal sensation with a skin pencil. This technique is particularly useful in evaluating patients with suspected lesions involving peripheral structures, in whom it will be necessary to distinguish between radiculopathies, plexopathies, and neuropathies. These distinctions are easily made by the examiner who has a solid grasp of peripheral neuroanatomy.

Pin testing may yield complete failure to perceive the stimulus; reduced perception; normal perception; or a heightened, perhaps unpleasant, perception. In cases of peripheral neuropathy, a patient may have areas of no sensation and reduced sensation in close relation to one another. Careful mapping of these findings with a skin pencil may be important for documentation of changes that may occur over time as a result of natural changes in the patient's condition or in response to therapeutic intervention.

Clinical observations associated with pin testing are documented qualitatively in the patient's chart and must include the patient's description of sensation in the area judged to be abnormal. The skin areas involved must be fully and completely described; it is frequently useful to make a simple drawing in the patient's record, illustrating the areas of sensory abnormality.

Lesions involving peripheral nerve structures produce the most clear-cut findings on sensory examination, although lesions involving CNS structures can also produce easily demonstrable sensory deficits to pin testing. Lesions that destroy or otherwise completely block transmission in postplexus peripheral nerves produce both anesthesia and analgesia in the cutaneous distribution of the nerve or nerves involved. Patients with such injuries do not perceive the pin stimulus when it is applied in these areas. Partial peripheral nerve injuries may produce reduced perception or exaggerated or distorted perceptions to pin stimuli, depending on the nature of the nerve injury. Individuals with reduced perception to noxious stimuli (hypalgesia) typically report the pin stimulus to be dull rather than sharp. Patients with enhanced perception to noxious stimuli (hyperalgesia) may report that the pin stimulus feels sharper or more unpleasant in the involved skin areas. Some patients may report peculiar sensations in an area of skin in the absence of any cutaneous stimulation. Frequently these sensations are likened to pins and needles or the sensation that a body part feels warmer or colder than usual. Unusual or abnormal cutaneous sensory experiences that are noticeable, annoying, or distracting but not necessarily unpleasant are referred to as *paresthesias*. Unpleasant or painful cutaneous sensory experiences are referred to as *dysesthesias*. The term *allodynia* describes a condition in which nonnoxious stimuli evoke the experience of pain.

Being unable to perceive the sharp noxious stimulus of a pin or perceiving it as dull can be seen in patients with lesions involving CNS structures, most notably the axons of the anterolateral tracts. Unilateral lesions involving these axons frequently result in the pin stimulus being perceived as dull on the contralateral side of the body, usually beginning one or two spinal segments below the level of the lesion. Diseases involving the subcortical white matter that damage thalamocortical projections from the ventral posterior nuclei to the primary sensory cortex frequently result in reduced perception to pin testing. The deficit will be evident on the contralateral side. Lesions involving the cerebral cortex usually leave the perception of the sharp stimulus essentially intact, but the ability to localize the site of application precisely may be impaired. Such a condition is known as *atopognosia*.

Complete testing requires that both sides of the body be evaluated. Comparisons between the two sides are particularly important when the history or other clinical findings suggest unilateral CNS involvement or peripheral nervous system disease. Sites proximal and distal on a limb should also be compared, inasmuch as some disease processes affect distal parts of peripheral nerves preferentially or before they affect more proximal parts of the nerve. Side-to-side asymmetries and differences in proximal versus distal sensation have important diagnostic and therapeutic implications.

Because of the possibility of puncturing the skin with the pin, it is necessary that a new, clean pin be used with each patient. The risk of infection is real and the cost of pins is negligible. The same pin should never be used on more than one patient.

Occasional patients willfully give false information when being tested. It may be possible to detect such behavior by asking the patient to say "yes" when the pin is felt and "no" when it is not. Be careful in deciding whether it is appropriate to use this tactic. This technique should not be used routinely, but it may be helpful when your index of suspicion is high.

In patients with unilateral disease involving the CNS, stimuli applied in the midline should be perceived as a result of the normal overlap of peripheral nerve fibers in the midline. In other patients, the ability to perceive the sharp stimulus may be reduced and the responses to pin stimulation may be inconsistent with repeated testing. To deal with these issues, some authors suggest that a correct response rate of at least 5 out of 5 should be used as evidence of intact sensory awareness.

Thermal Testing

Normal individuals should be able to recognize whether a stimulus applied to the skin is either hotter or colder than the skin and also to distinguish gradations in thermal sensation. Thermoreceptors in the skin are sensitive to changes in temperature and convey this information to the CNS along thinly myelinated (A_δ) and unmyelinated (C) peripheral nerve fibers. Transmission of nerve impulses to higher levels of the neuraxis is believed to occur by way of axons located in the anterolateral tracts.

Small glass vials or test tubes that can be filled with warm (50°C) or cold (10°C) water can be used for testing purposes. Care should be taken to keep the outside surfaces of the containers dry because, if the skin becomes wet, evaporation and cooling will result. Testing should be performed promptly after filling the containers, before the temperature of the liquid equilibrates with the room temperature.

Initially, each container should be brought in contact with the skin in an area known to be normal. This provides the patient with an opportunity to experience the thermal sensations about which he or she will be asked to make judgments during the actual testing. The patient should be asked to identify the stimulus as warm or cool, and the clinician must be sure that the patient is able to make these distinctions correctly.

When ready to begin, the patient should be instructed to close his or her eyes and respond by saying "warm" or "cool" immediately upon feeling the container applied to the skin. The examiner should apply the two stimuli, one at a time, in random order, beginning with the areas of skin suspected of being abnormal. Stimuli should also be delivered to normal areas of skin from time to time to ensure that the temperature of the water has not equilibrated to such a level that the patient can no longer distinguish warm from cool in normal areas.

Normal individuals should make no incorrect responses, provided that the stimuli are thermally adequate. Any incorrect responses can be judged as suggestive of a deficit in thermal sensibility. If a deficit is found, it is important to determine its boundaries precisely so that a decision can be made as to whether the lesion producing it is likely to involve peripheral or CNS structures. Deficits resulting from peripheral nerve lesions may be complete and clear-cut or partial. In either case, the clinician must judge whether the deficit suggests disease involving nerve roots, components of a nerve plexus, or postplexus peripheral nerves. Data derived from other motor and sensory tests may be helpful in this regard. The ability of the clinician to interpret test results correctly requires knowledge of peripheral neuroanatomy, specifically the cutaneous distribution of segmental and postplexus peripheral nerves (see Figs. 28 and 29).

Lesions involving the ALS are frequently associated with reductions in the ability to distinguish among different thermal stimuli applied to the skin. In the case of unilateral lesions involving the anterolateral tracts in the spinal cord, the deficit will be observed on the contralateral side and will be clearly demonstrable in areas at least two spinal segments below the level of the lesion. Thermal sensibility on the face in these patients will be intact. Lesions at the level of the mesencephalon or higher generally cause a contralateral deficit involving both the body and the face.

When tests of thermal sensibility are performed, the results should be documented in the patient's record. The note should indicate whether the patient had difficulty in distinguishing warm or cool temperatures, or both, and should precisely and completely describe the skin areas involved. A quantitative assessment can be included by indicating in ratio form the number of correct responses to either warm or cool stimuli over the number of trials. For example, testing may reveal six out of six correct responses to cool stimuli on the lateral surface of the right forearm and three out of six on the lateral surface of the left forearm. Such a finding would suggest a peripheral neuropathy involving the lateral antebrachial cutaneous nerve on the left side.

Thermal sensibility testing is somewhat cumbersome and may not be necessary in every patient complaining of a sensory problem. It is most useful in patients with suspected disease involving peripheral nervous system structures, in whom it will be important to determine the type of peripheral fibers involved and the exact location of the deficit-producing injury or disease process. Test results can often be valuable as a means of corroborating or reinforcing an impression derived from the history or previous testing.

Deep Pain

Deep pain, in the context of the neurologic examination, refers to the experience of discomfort originating from somatic structures beneath the skin, rather than from visceral organs such as the appendix. Generally included in this category are muscles, tendons, bone, fascia, bursae, and joints. Any of these structures can become injured or diseased and can give rise to the experience of pain. Nerve impulses associated with damage to these structures are thought to be transmitted to the CNS along thinly myelinated (A_δ) and unmyelinated (C) peripheral nerve fibers. Within the CNS, transmission to higher centers is thought to be by way of axons in the anterolateral tracts. Generally, perception of deep pain is tested only in patients who are in stupor or coma.

The ability to perceive deep pain is tested by applying a noxious stimulus to a subcutaneous structure. The easiest way of achieving this goal is by squeezing a body part. Manual pressure applied to the Achilles tendon or testicle can be used with ease and success in conscious individuals. It is useful to apply the stimulus to both sides equally and simultaneously and inquire as to whether the perceived discomfort was the same or different on the two sides. Some care must be taken to ensure that the stimulus is not so unpleasant that the patient is distracted by its magnitude and not able to judge whether the two experiences are the same or different. The report of test results should specify the stimulus used and indicate whether a difference was or was not perceived. If a difference was noted, the side demonstrating reduced pain sensation should be recorded. The test is contraindicated in patients with known pathology involving either the Achilles tendon or the testes.

Assessment of the Dorsal Column–Medial Lemniscus System

Light Touch

The ability to perceive light touch (*thigmesthesia*) is tested using tactile stimuli that activate low-threshold mechanoreceptors in the skin. These receptors are associated with myelinated (A_β) afferent nerve fibers, which conduct nerve impulses rapidly to the CNS. Within the CNS, nerve impulses are thought to be transmitted rostrally along axons of the dorsal column–medial lemniscus system, although conduction along the anterolateral tracts cannot be completely ruled out.

Areas of skin that should be tested include the foot, leg, thigh, trunk, hand, forearm, arm, and face. Skin in the distribution of specific peripheral nerves should be tested if specific peripheral neuropathy is suspected. The patient should be instructed to sit or lie comfortably and keep his or her eyes closed while being tested. Stimulation can be applied by means of a cotton wisp or a fine camel hair brush. The proper technique of applying the stimulus is to simply touch the skin lightly with the cotton wisp or brush. Do not drag or skim the stimulus along the skin, as this might cause movement of hairs on the skin which can be perceived (*trichoesthesia*) or may result in the sensation of tickle. The stimulus should be applied to a single spot on the skin, and the patient should be asked to respond immediately by saying "yes" if the stimulus is felt. It is wise to apply the stimulus to an area of skin where sensation is normal first to ensure that the patient can perceive the stimulus.

Stimulation should be delivered to comparable sites on both sides of the body and face, carefully noting the response on each side. Failure to detect the stimulus indicates reduced tactile sensitivity and suggests neurologic dysfunction. It is important to map out areas of reduced sensibility carefully and precisely so that judgments can be made regarding the anatomic location of a deficit-producing lesion. The examiner should note in the patient's record the distribution of sensory deficits and include a simple drawing of the hypesthetic area if necessary to ensure that the record is adequate. Testing with Von Frey monofilaments may be necessary if a quantitative record of light touch sensibility is needed.

The most common abnormality seen with testing for light touch is an inability to detect the stimulus (*thigmanesthesia*). Occasionally patients report light touch stimuli to be painful (*allodynia*).

Vibratory Sense

The ability to perceive vibratory stimuli (*pallesthesia*) is tested using a tuning fork that vibrates at a frequency of 128 Hz. The receptors activated by this stimulus are low-threshold, very rapidly adapting pacinian corpuscles located in the dermal layers of the skin. Although some writers view vibratory sense as a "deep" sensation, the location of the receptors activated by vibratory stimuli suggest rather that it is a "superficial" sense. The nerve impulses generated by the low-amplitude vibratory stimulus are transmitted along rapidly conducting A_β peripheral nerve fibers. Within the neuraxis, this information is thought to be carried by axons composing the dorsal column–medial lemniscus system.

Vibratory sense is tested by placing the base of a vibrating tuning fork against the skin, generally over a bony prominence. In this way, the low-amplitude movements of the tuning fork can be faithfully transmitted to the low-threshold, very rapidly adapting receptors, which are lightly compressed against the underlying bony structure. The tuning fork is set in motion by gently banging the tines against the examiner's hand while holding the fork near its base. Vibration should be of sufficient intensity to be felt initially and to come to a stop in about 10 to 15 seconds. Some practice is required to develop skill in setting the tines in motion equally each time.

The patient should be instructed to focus his or her attention on the vibration and not on the pressure of the tuning fork, and to respond by saying "stop" immediately when the experience of vibration can no longer be felt. Because the examiner is holding the tuning fork near its base, he or she will have a good indication of whether or not vibrations are still perceptible. Both sides of the body should be tested. Sites frequently used for this purpose include the great toe, malleoli, tibial tubercle, thumb, ulnar tubercle, medial humeral condyle, and the acromion process. Testing should begin distally on a limb, progressing to the more proximal sites.

Inability to perceive vibratory stimuli (*pallanesthesia*) or vibratory perception that extinguishes too quickly are suggestive of neurologic dysfunction involving either myelinated fibers in peripheral nerves or axons of the dorsal column–medial lemniscus system. Lesions involving peripheral nerve fibers or the axons located in the dorsal columns produce pallanesthesia on the ipsilateral side. Lesions in the brainstem or forebrain produce deficits on the contralateral side of the body. Therefore, precise localization of lesions associated with deficits in vibratory sense will require additional evidence of other sensory or motor abnormalities. Vibratory sense is rarely impaired in patients with lesions rostral to the thalamus.

The only deficit associated with vibratory testing is a decrease in sensitivity. The clinician should document the deficit by indicating the exact location and side on which a deficit is noted.

Position Sense

The ability to know where one's body parts are in space (*proprioception*) is an important requisite for motor function. It is likely that the nervous system monitors joint position to achieve this goal, and in that regard, muscle spindles and joint receptors are the receptors most likely to be involved. Transmission of impulses to the CNS occurs by way of large, myelinated peripheral nerve fibers (Ia, II and A_β) associated with these various receptors. Most authors argue that information about position sense is relayed to higher brain centers along axons of the dorsal column–medial lemniscus system, although recently the role of this system in position sense has been questioned.

The patient should be positioned comfortably in the sitting or lying position and instructed to keep his or her eyes closed while being tested. The test procedure involves moving a toe or finger through a small range of flexion and extension. Proper technique is essential if reliable results are to be obtained. The examiner must grasp the digit by placing his or her fingers on its lateral surfaces in such a way that only one joint will be moved in the plane of flexion and extension. The digit must not be grasped on its dorsal and ventral sides because movement will cause a change in pressure on one of these surfaces that is easily detected by the patient and involves receptors other than those that are responsive to joint position. The examiner should move the joint slightly into either flexion or extension and the patient should be instructed to respond immediately, indicating whether the digit moved "up" or "down." It is not necessary to move the joint through its full range of motion. In fact, doing so may activate other receptors that may invalidate test results. Only a small degree of movement is necessary to elicit a response. The patient should be asked to respond to the position of the joint relative to its starting or previous position. A response from the patient should be elicited when the movement has stopped, not while the joint is being moved, since the examiner is interested in position sense (proprioception) rather than movement sense (*kinesthesia*). Movements into flexion and extension should be in random order, and the patient should be asked to respond to at least six or seven placements.

Neurologically intact individuals should make no mistakes in responding to whether the joint is "up" or "down" relative to the previous position. Any errors suggest neurologic dysfunction. Peripheral nerve or spinal cord lesions result in ipsilateral deficits, whereas lesions in the brainstem or cerebrum cause deficits on the contralateral side. Fingers and toes should be tested bilaterally and comparisons made of the responses on both sides. The chart record should indicate in ratio form the number of correct responses versus the number of trials for each digit tested. For example, the report for a normal individual would read: proprioception—seven out of seven correct responses for the left great toe.

Assessment of Cortical Sensory Function

Traced Figure Identification

The ability to recognize and identify numbers or letters written on the skin (*graphesthesia*) requires a functionally intact parietal lobe. More specifically, the parietal association areas are thought to be necessary for this function. Individuals who have intact graphesthesia are presumed to be without neurologic disease involving peripheral afferent fibers, the ascending spinal pathways, or the parietal lobes. However, patients who are unable to recognize traced figures (*graphagnosia*) may or may not have other somatic sensory deficits. Patients who demonstrate unilateral graphagnosia in the absence of other somatic sensory deficits are likely to have lesions involving the contralateral parietal association cortices or the immediate underlying white matter.

Clinical tests for graphesthesia are usually performed on the palm of the hand, although other skin areas can be used. The examiner should extend the patient's arm forward, with the elbow extended, forearm pronated, and wrist extended such that the palm of the patient's hand is vertical, facing away, with the fingers pointing up. In this position, the examiner will be able to scribe a letter or number on the palm without the patient being able to see what is being written. In addition, because the fingers are pointed up, the orientation of the letter or number written on the palm will be similar to what it would be if the patient were to scribe it himself or herself while looking at the palm. The examiner should explain to the patient what will be done and instruct him or her to respond by naming the letter or number that is written on the palm. The examiner should exert an even force, scribing the letter or number over the full extent of the palm. The speed should be such that the writing requires about one full second. Numbers 3, 4, and 6, and letters A, B, and C are useful because they are sufficiently different from one another and are easily recognized by most individuals.

Graphagnosia should be documented in the patient's record by indicating the side on which it is found and the letters or numbers used. Both sides should always be tested. Generally, patients who demonstrate graphagnosia also demonstrate some other abnormality of cortical sensory function.

Object Identification

The ability to recognize and identify objects based on their tactile characteristics (*stereognosis*), like traced figure identification, requires a functionally intact parietal association cortex. Individuals in whom stereognosis is intact are not likely to have deficits to pin testing, thigmanesthesia, or pallanesthesia, or to have impaired proprioception, but patients with one or more of these deficits, particularly thigmanesthesia and impaired proprioception, are likely to have difficulty with object identification (*astereognosis*). Patients who demonstrate unilateral astereognosis in the absence of other somatic sensory deficits are likely to have disease involving the contralateral parietal association cortices or the immediately underlying white matter.

Tests for stereognosis involve asking the patient to identify common, everyday objects by touch without looking at them. Test objects should be small enough to be held and manipulated with one hand. Objects that are easy to obtain and convenient to use include coins, safety pins, paper clips, and keys. When performing tests for stereognosis, it is important to ensure that the patient cannot see the objects that he or she is being asked to identify. In addition, the objects should be handled in such a way that they do not make noise; otherwise, the patient may be given an auditory clue as to their identity.

Both sides of the body should be tested, and the patient's record should indicate the objects used, stating clearly which objects were identified correctly and incorrectly. Generally, correct responses using two or three objects is sufficient to judge stereognosis to be intact.

Double Simultaneous Stimulation

The ability to perceive two identical stimuli applied simultaneously to corresponding areas on both sides of the body requires a certain level of cortical attention. Neurologically intact individuals, when stimulated this way, report an awareness of both stimuli. Patients with disease involving the parietal lobe will perceive the stimulus only on one side, or initially may report perceiving both stimuli but quickly come to perceive it only on one side. In such cases, the side on which the stimulus is not felt or on which it becomes extinguished will be the side contralateral to the parietal lobe dysfunction.

Tests for double simultaneous stimulation are usually performed on the face, arms, and legs. The patient should be instructed to close his or her eyes and respond by saying "right," "left," or "both" to indicate the side or sides where the touch stimuli are felt. The examiner should lightly touch corresponding areas on both sides of the face, arms, or legs with equal intensity and duration. The touches should not be perceived as painful. It is essential that the tactile stimuli delivered to each side be identical in every respect. Failure to adhere to this last admonition will bias the patient toward the more prominent stimulus and result in an unreliable test result.

The test results should be reported by indicating the skin areas tested and on which side, if either, extinction was demonstrated. Caution in interpreting test results is warranted in patients who are not alert, who are inattentive, or who for some other reason are unable to fully cooperate with the examiner's request.

SUMMARY

The evaluation of sensory function in patients with complaints of sensory abnormality or loss can be difficult. Much of the difficulty stems from the subjective nature of sensory experience and the limited and sometimes inadequate ways that exist for describing sensory abnormalities. Accurate and reliable testing requires knowledge and skill in the methods of evaluation and experience in the interpretation of clinical findings. An important requirement also is the ability to listen carefully and respectfully to the patient, who may be struggling to communicate essential features of an uncomfortable, perhaps new, and possibly frightening experience. Thoughtful practice and attention to detail will help ensure the accuracy and reliability of the results of sensory evaluation.

RECORDING AND PRESENTING DATA

*T*his section consists of forms that can be used for making notes while performing the neurologic examination, and a suggested order for presenting the collected data. The format presented here is comprehensive in scope, reflecting the author's view that it is necessary to learn how to perform a complete and thorough examination before it is possible to use a less detailed version effectively. Inexperienced clinicians must acquire skill and competence in performing all tests and measures that compose the neurologic examination before they can consider themselves competent in neurologic evaluation. Practice and experience bring knowledge and wisdom, and these form the basis for being able to tailor the neurologic examination to the individual needs of the patient and the clinical situation.

INTERVIEW AND HISTORY

Name (initials) ———————————— ID# ——————————

Date of Birth — / — / — Age ——— Place of Birth ———————

Sex ————— Race ————— Religion ——————————

Residence (city, state) ——————————————————————

Marital Status: Single ——— Married ——— Divorced ——— Widowed ———

Hand Used for Writing: Right ——— Left ———

Chief Complaint (CC)

History of Present Illness (HPI)
(date and manner of onset, setting at onset, location, quality, severity, duration, frequency, precipitating or aggravating factors, remissions and exacer-
bations, alleviating factors, relevant negative information, relevant family information, associated phenomena)

Past Medical History (PMH)

(birth circumstances, childhood illnesses, previous adult illnesses, past hospitalizations including dates and problems, transfusions, past injuries or accidents, previous surgery)

Pertinent Health Information

Allergies (drug, environmental, food, other)

Immunizations (tetanus, polio, influenza, Hepatavax, Pneumovax)

Habits (tobacco, alcohol, abuse drugs)

Medications (name, dose, frequency, date started)

Screening tests (blood pressure, cholesterol, tuberculin, urinary analysis)

Cancer tests (skin, colon, prostate, breast, Pap, etc.)

Sleep patterns

Appetite, diet, eating habits

Sexual habits

Family History (FH)
(parents, siblings, spouse, children, pertinent relatives: age, health, or age at and cause of death)

Social History (SH)
(relationships, residence, travel, exercise and leisure activities, educational level, economic status)

Occupational History (OH)
(employment status, work activities and level of satisfaction, previous work, other work training, military experience)

Review of Systems (ROS)

General (usual state of health, chills, fever, sweats, fatigue, malaise, weight change)

Skin (lesions, dryness, color, temperature, texture, petechiae, odor, hives, masses, itching, bruises, rash, moles, pigmentation, nails, hair, cancer)

HEENT
general (pain, stiffness, swelling; describe location and characteristics)

eyes (corrective lenses, pain, visual loss, diplopia, dryness, tearing, infections, photophobia, redness, blurring, flashing lights, visual distortions, illusions, cataracts, glaucoma)

ears (hearing aids, pain, deafness, tinnitus, infections, discharge, trauma)

nose and sinuses (colds, pain, obstruction, discharge, infection, sneezing, anosmia, bleeding, peculiar odors) mouth and throat (dentition, pain, gums, bleeding, swelling, dryness, dysphagia, salivation, peculiar tastes, dysphonia, lesions, odor)

neck (pain, tenderness, swelling, stiffness, node enlargement)

Breasts (masses, dimples, discharge, pain, asymmetry)

Respiratory (cough, dyspnea, hemoptysis, sputum, wheezing, stridor, orthopnea, cyanosis, crackles, asthma, pneumonia, emphysema, exercise limits, occupational exposure)

Cardiac (angina, murmur, palpitations, hypertension, infarction, conduction block, rheumatic fever, orthopnea, syncope, paroxysmal nocturnal dyspnea, exercise limitations)

Vascular (pulses, varicosities, ulcers, claudication, phlebitis)

Gastrointestinal (abdominal pain or distension, thirst, appetite, anorexia, nausea, vomiting, indigestion, jaundice, ulcers, belching, hernia, hepatitis, hematemesis, hemorrhoids, rectal bleeding or discomfort, constipation, diarrhea, flatulence, incontinence, bowel habits, laxative use)

Renal and urinary (anuria, dysuria, enuresis, flank pain, suprapubic pain, frequency, urgency, hematuria, nocturia, incontinence, oliguria, polyuria, pyuria, stones, infection, changes in color or odor, renal disease)

Gynecologic (menarche, menopause, cycle length, menorrhagia, metrorrhagia, amenorrhea, pelvic pain, dysmenorrhea, spotting, discharge, pruritus, tumor, dyspareunia, venereal disease, contraceptive use, pregnancies, live births, stillbirths, abortions)

Male genitalia (pain, swelling, discharge, skin lesions, itch, venereal disease, potency, prostate)

Musculoskeletal (pain, cramps, stiffness, swelling, motion limitation, fractures, trauma, temperature changes, discoloration, backache, arthritis)

Neurologic (pain, headache, syncope, memory, confusion, cognition, disorientation, dizziness, mood changes, speech, dysphagia, seizures, spasms, tremor, twitching, weakness, paralyses, sensory changes, coordination, visual or hearing changes, gait disturbances, anosmia, abnormal movements)

Endocrine (weight change, temperature tolerance, changes in eating or drinking, secondary sex changes, fatigue, diabetes, goiter, exophthalmos)

Hematopoietic (anemia, bleeding, bruising, exposure to radiation, blood type)

Psychiatric (anxiety, insomnia, hallucinations, depression, guilt, mood swings, past psychiatric problems)

Reliability of historical information _____

EXAMINATIONS

General Appearance
(hygiene, level of distress, appearance relative to chronologic age, attitude, mobility status, communication)

Vital Signs

BP (position) ——————— RUE ——————— LUE ———————

Temp ——————— HR ——————— RR ———————

Ht ——————— Wt ———————

General Physical Examination

Integument
skin (scars, bruises, rash, telangiectasia, texture, pigmentation, turgor, petechiae, nodules, ulcers, jaundice, blisters, tumors)

nails (clubbing, color, nail bed)

hair (distribution, texture, scalp)

Lymph Nodes (cervical, auricular, occipital, supraclavicular, axillary, epitrochlear, inguinal: size, fixed, mobile, firm, matted, tender)

Head (skull shape, tenderness, defects, bruits)

Eyes (exophthalmos, ptosis, scleral hemorrhages, icterus, conjunctival injection or petechiae, cornea, arcus senilis, strabismus, anisocoria, acuity)

Ears (discharge, tympanic membrane, auricle, mastoid)

Nose (shape, obstruction, congestion, discharge, polyps, septum, sinus tenderness, lesions)

Mouth and Throat
  general (hygiene, odor, salivary glands)

lips (color, sores, pigmentation, cyanosis, cheilosis)

teeth (dentures, number, condition)

gingiva (color, ulcers, pigmentation, periodontal disease)

tongue (atrophy, color, deviation, ulcers, tremor, masses)

pharynx (tonsils, color, exudates, uvula position, palatal movements)

Neck
general (mobility, masses, tenderness, swelling)

vessels (arterial pulsations, venous engorgement, bruits)

thyroid (size, nodules)

trachea (position, mobility)

Breasts (symmetry, masses, pigmentation, nipples, tenderness, dimpling, secretions)

Chest and lungs (symmetry, shape, respiratory excursion, diameters, tactile fremitus, diaphragmatic movement, resonance, breath sounds, wheezes, crackles, friction rub, bronchophony, pectoriloquy)

Heart (visible pulsations, apical impulse, precordial bulge, thrills, precordial heave, rate, rhythm, heart sounds, rubs, clicks, murmurs, gallops)

Abdomen (visible asymmetry, palpable organs, tenderness, spasm, hernias, rebound, guarding, rigidity, masses, tympany, bowel sounds, fluid waves, peristalsis)

Genitalia
  male (development, pubic hair, circumcision, urethral strictures, testes, epididymis, varicocele, hydrocele, edema, urethral discharge, skin lesions, testicular pain or masses)

female (development, pubic hair, clitoris, urethra, introitus, prolapse, cervix, discharge, masses, tenderness, lesions)

Anus and rectum (sphincter tone, hemorrhoids, fissures, fistulae, prostate, masses, stool guaiac, lesions, tenderness, bleeding, incontinence)

Limbs (deformities, color, sweating, dryness, joint inflammation, pain or tenderness, edema, atrophy, contractures, ulcers, varicosities, amputations, temperature, movement limitations)

Peripheral pulses (strong, weak, thready, absent)

	Right	Left
radial	_____	_____
femoral	_____	_____
popliteal	_____	_____
posterior tibial	_____	_____
dorsal pedes	_____	_____

Back and spine (posture, curvatures, mobility, tenderness, nerve root pain, meningismus)

Neurologic Examination

Mental Status
level of consciousness
alert   lethargic   obtunded   stupor   coma
attention
attentive   fluctuating   inattentive
orientation ($\times 3$, $\times 2$, $\times 1$)
person _____ place _____ time _____

language (native _____ acquired _____)
mute

spontaneous speech (intact/impaired)
prosody
dysphonia
dysarthria (K   L   M)

fluency (intact/impaired—stuttering/stammering)
number of words per minute _____

comprehension (intact/impaired)

repetition (intact/impaired)
(indicate words or phrases used)

naming and word finding (intact/impaired)
(indicate words used)

reading and writing (intact/impaired)

learning and memory
recent (intact/impaired)

words recalled _____ elapsed time _____
short story recall

items in story _____

number recalled _____

digit span _____
long-term (intact/impaired)

past presidents: number recalled _____
other evidence (describe)

cognitive and cortical function
fund of knowledge (appropriate/limited)

calculation (intact/impaired)
(indicate test used—serial 7's, 3's, other)

proverb interpretation (intact/impaired)
(indicate proverb used)

gnosia
visual (intact/impaired)
(indicate object used)

auditory (intact/impaired)
(indicate sound used)

finger (intact/impaired)

praxis
buccofacial (intact/impaired)
(indicate task)

limb (intact/impaired)
(indicate task)

trunk (intact/impaired)
(indicate task)

constructional (intact/impaired)
(indicate task)

mood and affect (characterize)
   appropriate
   inappropriate

thought content
   coherent, organized
   incoherent, disorganized, paranoid, other

Cranial Nerves
  I. Olfactory (intact/impaired)
    (indicate odors used)

    R ——————— L ———————

  II. Optic
     visual acuity   OD   OS

       uncorrected   ——————   ——————

       corrected   ——————   ——————
     visual fields
       (full, restricted)

                            OD   OS

      describe field defect ————————————————————
     light reflex (intact/impaired)   OD   OS

       direct   —————— ——————

       indirect   —————— ——————
     swinging flashlight test (intact/impaired)
       (if impaired, describe findings)

accommodation (near) reflex (intact/impaired)
(if impaired, describe findings)

fundus (disk, vessels, optic cup, macula, color, size)
(describe observations including papilledema, optic atrophy, vessel nicking, drusen)

III. Oculomotor, IV trochlear, VI abducens

	Right	Left
palpebral fissures (height)	——	——
ptosis	——	——
pupils (diameter in ambient light) (normal, miosis, corectasia)	——	——

tests in position of primary gaze
   corneal light reflex   (normal, abnormal)
   red glass test   (normal, diplopia)
   Maddox rod   (normal, diplopia)
   cover-uncover test   (normal, abnormal)
   ocular deviation

	OD	OS
heterotropia		
esotropia	——	——
exotropia	——	——
hypertropia	——	——
hypotropia	——	——
heterophoria		
esophoria	——	——
exophoria	——	——
hyperphoria	——	——
hypophoria	——	——
extraocular movements (tracking)	OD	OS
abduction	——	——
abduction with elevation	——	——

abduction with depression   _____   _____

adduction   _____   _____

adduction with elevation   _____   _____

adduction with depression   _____   _____
(describe positions of *maximal* and *minimal* diplopia)

extraocular movements (volitional)	OD	OS
abduction	_____	_____
abduction with elevation	_____	_____
abduction with depression	_____	_____
adduction	_____	_____
adduction with elevation	_____	_____
adduction with depression	_____	_____

(describe movements that *maximize* and *minimize* diplopia)

Indicate recognized abnormalities (i.e., internuclear ophthalmo-plegia, Horner's syndrome, Argyll Robertson pupil, Adie's pupil, Marcus Gunn pupil, miosis, corectasia, iridoplegia, cycloplegia, proptosis).

V. Trigeminal
sensory (intact, absent, reduced, paresthesia, dysesthesia)

	Right	Left
corneal reflex	_____	_____
ophthalmic nerve	_____	_____
maxillary nerve	_____	_____
mandibular nerve	_____	_____

motor (normal, weak, absent)

masseter   _____   _____

temporalis   _____   _____

enunciation (em em em, bee bee bee, pee pee pee)

VII. Facial

	Right	Left
sensory-taste (intact/impaired) (indicate test substance used.)	_____	_____

motor (intact, weak, absent)	Right	Left
frontalis	_____	_____
orbicularis oculi	_____	_____
zygomaticus	_____	_____
orbicularis oris	_____	_____
platysma	_____	_____
lacrimation	_____	_____

VIII. Vestibulocochlear   Right   Left

cochlear nerve

	Right	Left
finger rubbing (distance)	_____	_____
Rinne (AC:BC)	_____	_____
Weber (lateralizes to)	_____	_____

vestibular nerve

	Right	Left
past-pointing test (drift to the)	_____	_____
marching in place (rotation to the)	_____	_____
gaze nystagmus (gaze to)	_____	_____

Nylen-Bárány test

Head rotation to R (nystagmus, vertigo, nausea)

Head rotation to L (nystagmus, vertigo, nausea)

caloric testing (cold water)	Right	Left
right ear		
nystagmus to	_____	_____
past-pointing to	_____	_____

left ear

    nystagmus to   ‾‾‾‾‾‾‾   ‾‾‾‾‾‾‾

    past-pointing to   ‾‾‾‾‾‾‾   ‾‾‾‾‾‾‾

IX. Glossopharyngeal, X. Vagus
    position of uvula (midline, displaced R or L)
    soft palate (symmetric, lower on R or L)
    response to phonation
        (describe movement of uvula and soft palate)

    enunciation (kay kay kay)
    gag reflex (intact/absent)

XI. Spinal accessory	Right	Left
sternocleidomastoid (0–5)	‾‾‾‾‾	‾‾‾‾‾
trapezius (0–5)	‾‾‾‾‾	‾‾‾‾‾

XII. Hypoglossal	Right	Left
atrophy (yes/no)	‾‾‾‾‾	‾‾‾‾‾
fibrillations (yes/no)	‾‾‾‾‾	‾‾‾‾‾

deviation upon protrusion (midline, right, left)
enunciation (la la la, tee tee tee, dee dee dee)

Motor systems
    observable findings (atrophy, hypertrophy, bulk, contour, symmetry, fasciculations, abnormal movements)

girth measurements	Right	Left
arm	‾‾‾‾‾	‾‾‾‾‾
forearm	‾‾‾‾‾	‾‾‾‾‾
thigh	‾‾‾‾‾	‾‾‾‾‾
leg	‾‾‾‾‾	‾‾‾‾‾

muscle tone (decreased, normal, increased, spasticity, rigidity)
    (describe affected muscle groups)

muscle strength (0–5)	Right	Left
shoulder abduction	————	————
shoulder retraction	————	————
shoulder protraction	————	————
shoulder flexion	————	————
shoulder external rotation	————	————
shoulder internal rotation	————	————
elbow flexion	————	————
elbow extension	————	————
forearm supination	————	————
forearm pronation	————	————
wrist extension	————	————
wrist flexion	————	————
finger extension	————	————
finger flexion	————	————
finger abduction	————	————
finger adduction	————	————
grip strength	————	————
hip flexion	————	————
hip extension	————	————
hip abduction	————	————
hip adduction	————	————
knee extension	————	————
knee flexion	————	————
ankle dorsiflexion	————	————
ankle plantar flexion	————	————
pronator drift	————	————
heel walking	————————————	
toe walking	————————————	

coordination (normal, ataxic)	Right	Left
finger to nose	————	————
rebound phenomenon	————	————
supinate/pronate	————	————
finger tap	————	————
heel to shin	————	————
figure 8	————	————
toe tap	————	————

station and gait
    Romberg's test (positive, negative)
    gait (normal, ataxic, circumducted, festinating, steppage,   antalgic)
    tandem walking (normal, ataxic)

Reflexes (0–5)

muscle stretch	Right	Left
scapulohumeral	————	————
pectoral	————	————
deltoid	————	————
biceps brachii	————	————
brachioradialis	————	————
triceps	————	————
finger flexor	————	————
quadriceps femoris	————	————
adductor	————	————
hamstring	————	————
Achilles tendon	————	————

abnormal (present, absent)

jaw	————————————
snout	————————————
glabellar	————————————
Hoffmann's sign	————————————

cutaneous (intact, absent, abnormal)	Right	Left
abdominal upper	————	————

abdominal lower   _____   _____

cremasteric   _____   _____

bulbocavernosus   _____   _____

anal sphincter   _____   _____

plantar   _____   _____

abnormal (present, absent)

  Babinski's response   _____   _____

  palmomental   _____   _____

  palmar grasp   _____   _____

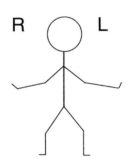

Sensory Systems

pin prick (intact, reduced, absent)

	Right	Left
hand	_____	_____
forearm	_____	_____
arm	_____	_____
thigh	_____	_____
leg	_____	_____
foot	_____	_____
face	_____	_____

(describe affected area and findings)

thermal sensation (intact, reduced, absent)

	Right	Left
hand	_____	_____
forearm	_____	_____
arm	_____	_____
thigh	_____	_____
leg	_____	_____
foot	_____	_____
face	_____	_____

(describe affected area and findings)

deep pain (intact, reduced, absent, hyperalgesia)

	Right	Left
Achilles tendon	_____	_____
testicle	_____	_____
other	_____	_____

light touch (intact, reduced, absent, hyperesthesia)

	Right	Left
hand	_____	_____
forearm	_____	_____
arm	_____	_____
thigh	_____	_____
leg	_____	_____
foot	_____	_____
face	_____	_____

(describe affected area and findings)

vibratory (intact, impaired)

	Right	Left
great toe	————	————
malleolus	————	————
tibial tubercle	————	————
thumb	————	————
ulnar tubercle	————	————
humeral condyle	————	————
acromion process	————	————

position sense (intact, impaired)

	Right	Left
finger	————	————
toe	————	————

cortical sensory function (intact, impaired)

	Right	Left
traced figure identification	————	————

(indicate numbers and letters used)

	Right	Left
object identification	————	————

(indicate objects used)

double simultaneous stimulation

	Right	Left
hand	————	————
forearm	————	————
arm	————	————
thigh	————	————
leg	————	————
foot	————	————
face	————	————

NEUROLOGIC PATIENT DATA PRESENTATION

General Information
    name, age, handedness, race, sex
    signs of distress or abnormality
    site of examination (bedside, clinic, emergency department)
    mobility status (bed, wheelchair, ambulatory)
Chief complaint(s)
History of present illness
Past medical history
Pertinent health information
Family history
Social history
Occupational history
Review of systems
Physical examination
    general appearance
    vital signs
    physical findings
Neurologic examination
    mental status
    cranial nerves
    motor systems and coordination
    reflexes
    sensory systems
Assessment and summary
Plan

SUMMARY OF THE NEUROLOGIC EXAMINATION

Mental Status

level of consciousness
attention
orientation
language function
 spontaneous speech
 fluency
 comprehension
 repetition
 naming and word finding
 reading and writing
learning and memory
 recent
 long-term
cognitive and cortical function
 fund of knowledge
 calculation
 proverb interpretation
 gnosia
 praxis
mood and affect
thought content

Cranial Nerves

olfactory
optic
 visual acuity

visual fields
light reflexes
accommodation reflex
funduscopic examination
oculomotor, trochlear, abducens
    palpebral fissures (ptosis)
    pupils
    ocular movements
        tracking
        volitional
trigeminal
    sensory
        corneal reflex
        ophthalmic, maxillary, mandibular nerves
    motor
        strength
        enunciation
facial
    sensory (taste)
    motor
        facial muscles
        lacrimation
vestibulocochlear
    cochlear
        finger rubbing
        Rinne
        Weber
    vestibular
        past-pointing
        marching in place
        gaze nystagmus
        Nylen-Bárány
        caloric testing
glossopharyngeal, vagus
    movements of uvula and soft palate
    gag reflex
    enunciation
spinal accessory
    sternocleidomastoid and trapezius
hypoglossal
    atrophy
    fibrillations
    deviation on protrusion
    enunciation

Motor Systems

observable findings
girth measurements
muscle tone
muscle strength
coordination
station and gait
    Romberg's test
    free walking
    tandem walking

Reflexes

muscle stretch
abnormal muscle stretch
cutaneous
abnormal cutaneous

Sensory Systems

pin prick
thermal sense
deep pain
light touch
vibratory sense
position sense
cortical sensory function
    traced figure identification (graphesthesia)
    object identification (stereognosis)
    double simultaneous stimulation (extinction)

INDEX

Numbers followed by an "f" indicate figures; numbers followed by a "t" indicate tables.

213